Dedicated to Jenifer, my loving wife;
Niyaash, my son, the joy of my life;
and Malcom and Kashmira, my dear parents,
for their unwavering support.

ECG QUICK START

A Practical Guide to Interpretation

DR. YAZAD MADAN

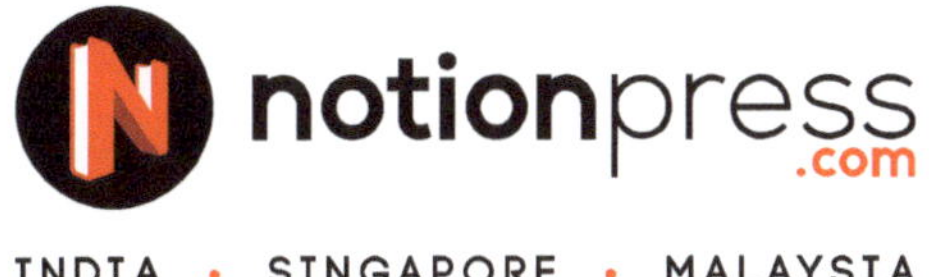

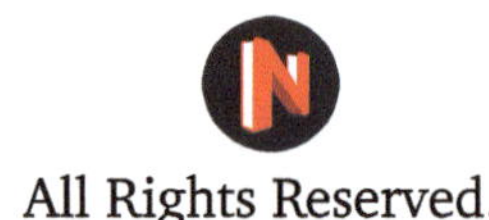

ISBN
Hardcase 979-8-89588-373-0
Paperback 979-8-89556-835-4

This book provides essential tools for basic ECG interpretation. While the methods are effective for most cases, ECG interpretation can be complex, and rare patterns may require specialized knowledge. Use this book as a starting point and consult experienced clinicians for definitive diagnoses. Note that certain analogies involving gender-based terms and relationships are used to clarify and explain concepts. These analogies are for illustrative purposes only and do not reflect any gender-based stereotypes or biases.

CONTENTS

FOREWORD

I am greatly honoured to write the foreword for this amazing book titled *ECG QUICK START: A Practical Guide to Interpretation*. In addition to containing a vast fund of knowledge, this book has been written in a clear, concise, and easily readable manner, enabling any medical professional to comprehend and appreciate its content.

I have enjoyed going through each of the chapters, which cover practically all important topics of ECG. The first chapter begins with an overview of leads and their importance, followed by the essential steps to read and interpret an ECG. It nicely elaborates on tachyarrhythmias (Atrial Fibrillation, Atrial Flutter, Supraventricular Tachycardia, Ventricular Tachycardia, and Polymorphic Ventricular Tachycardia) and bradyarrhythmias (Sinus Bradycardia, First-degree Heart Block, Second-degree Type I & II Heart Block, and Complete/Third-degree Heart Block). These topics have all been covered extensively with a stepwise approach and colour illustrations to facilitate easy understanding.

I would like to compliment and congratulate the author, Dr. Yazad Madan, for his hard work and dedication. This book will prove very useful for healthcare providers and practitioners of medicine. At every step, the author has taken great care to highlight the key features necessary to correctly identify rhythms, which can then be treated appropriately.

In this respect, the book goes beyond being just a medical treatise and serves as a guiding light for healthcare professionals. Knowledge is empowerment, and with the wealth of information available in this book, I am confident that the reader will be well-equipped to understand and educate others on the basics of ECG. I am sure that this book will have a wide circulation and achieve its goal of improving healthcare within the community.

Dr. Ketan Patel
FEM (UK), MRCEM (UK), FACEE, EBCEM
Consultant & Head, Dept. of Emergency Medicine
Programme Director - EM Residency
Zydus Hospitals & Healthcare Research Pvt Ltd
Ahmedabad, Gujarat, India

PREFACE

The year was 2020. The world was grappling with the COVID-19 pandemic, and India was no exception. Strict lockdowns brought a sharp decline in patient flow to hospitals. As a resident in Emergency Medicine, this unexpected downtime could have meant a pause in our academic pursuits. However, Dr. Ketan Patel, our esteemed mentor, had other plans. He believed this was an opportunity to delve deeper into the fascinating world of ECGs.

"Imagine you're writing a book on ECGs. What would you include?" Dr. Patel posed this challenge, igniting my curiosity. I spent months studying textbooks, articles, and guidelines, unraveling the complexities of ECGs. With Dr. Patel's guidance, I distilled this knowledge into a practical guide.

Applying this learning in real-world settings showed remarkable results. ECG interpretation, once a daunting task, became a process I could navigate with ease and speed.

After residency, I started teaching ECG interpretation. The reception was overwhelming but the feedback revealed a common struggle: the difficulty of recalling specific principles when applying them in practice.

This book is the answer to that need. It's not just a textbook, but a practical guide, designed for medical professionals – especially those new to ECG interpretation – to bridge the gap between theory and application.

Within these pages, you'll find a clear, concise approach, enriched with real-world scenarios and practical tips. My aim is to empower you to interpret ECGs with confidence, ultimately leading to better patient care.

Join me on this journey through ECG interpretation. Together, let's uncover its secrets.

Dr. Yazad Madan

INTRODUCTION

The electrocardiogram (ECG) is a fundamental tool for assessing heart function, yet mastering its interpretation can seem daunting. This book, **ECG Quick Start**, adopts a practical approach, equipping you with the essential skills to interpret basic ECGs, similar to how drivers navigate safely without needing to be mechanics.

Just as understanding the core functions of the gas pedal, brake, and steering wheel allows you to control your car effectively, this book focuses on identifying key features on an ECG that reflect the heart's electrical activity. By the end, you'll gain the confidence to interpret basic ECGs, contributing to informed clinical decisions and improved patient care.

This book serves as the first step in a comprehensive three-part series on ECG interpretation:

- ECG Quick Start (this book): Provides a foundation in interpreting basic ECGs.

- ECG Foundations: Delves into the underlying physiological principles of ECG formation.

- ECG Mastery: Refines your interpretation skills for tackling complex ECGs.

Whether you're a medical professional seeking a refresher or a complete beginner, this series provides a structured path to mastering ECG interpretation.

Here's what sets this book apart:

- Practical Focus: Prioritizes actionable skills for interpreting basic ECGs.

- Clear Explanations: Breaks down complex concepts into easily understandable terms.

- Structured Learning: Provides a foundational framework for further study.

Get ready to unlock the world of ECG interpretation with confidence!

LEADS

The ECG isn't just a squiggly line; it's a detailed picture of the heart's electrical activity.

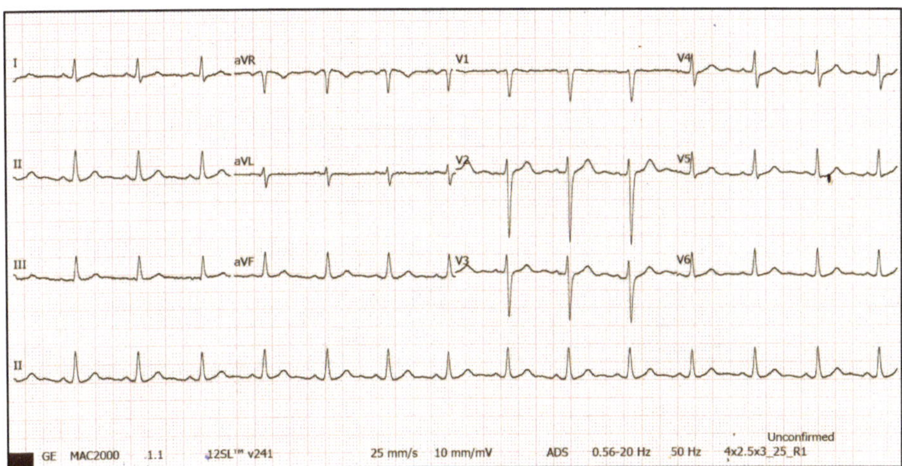

The **10 electrodes** are strategically placed, **1 on each limb and 6 over the chest** to form the **12 leads**. These leads act like eyes, providing different views of the heart's electrical activity.

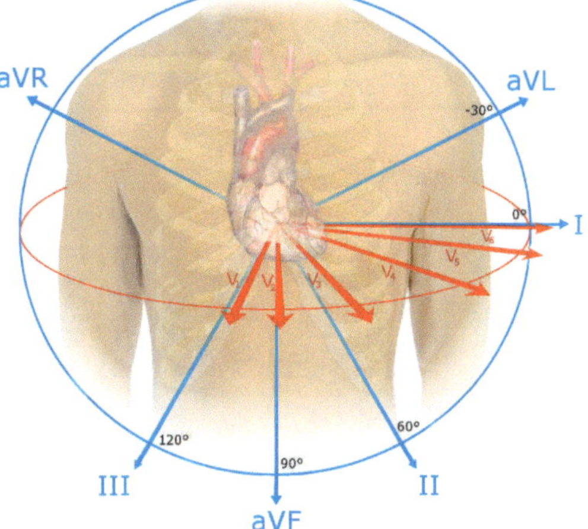

Limb Leads (I, II, III, aVR, aVL, aVF): These 6 leads use limb electrodes to view the heart's electrical activity from the side (**vertical plane**).

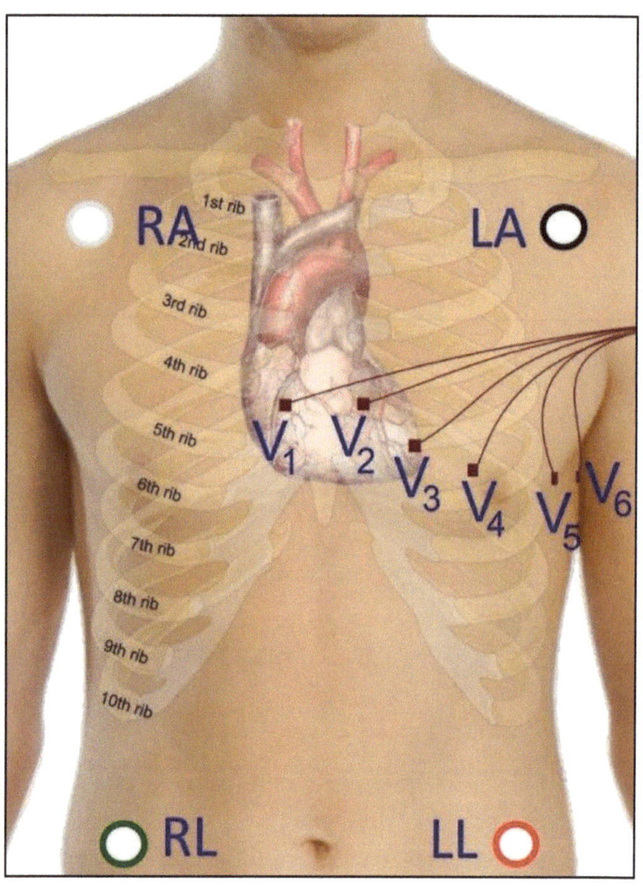

Chest Leads (V1-V6): These 6 leads use chest electrodes to view the heart's electrical activity from the front **(horizontal plane)**.

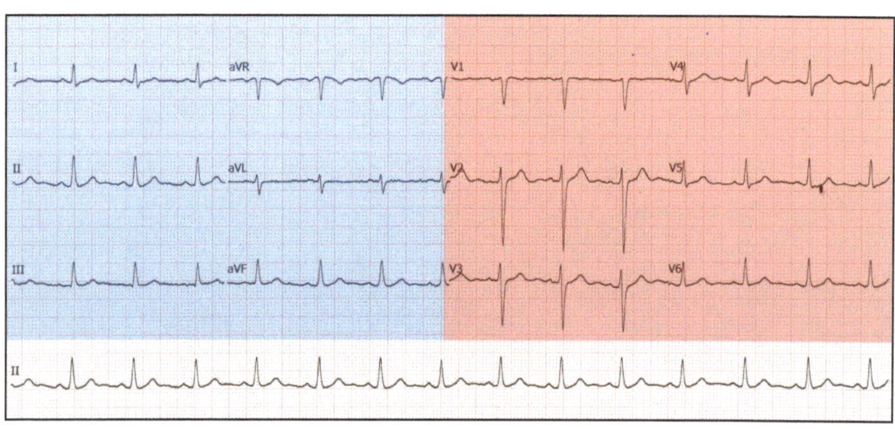

Before interpreting the ECG, we need to understand the basic building blocks of an ECG waveform. This waveform comprises 3 principal waves:

- **P Wave:** This deflection represents the electrical impulse initiating the depolarization (electrical activation) and subsequent contraction of the atria, the heart's upper chambers.

- **QRS Complex:** This group of waves signifies the depolarization of the ventricles (the lower pumping chambers), triggering their subsequent contraction.

- **T Wave:** This wave reflects ventricular repolarization (electrical recovery), indicating the ventricles are relaxing and preparing for the subsequent beat.

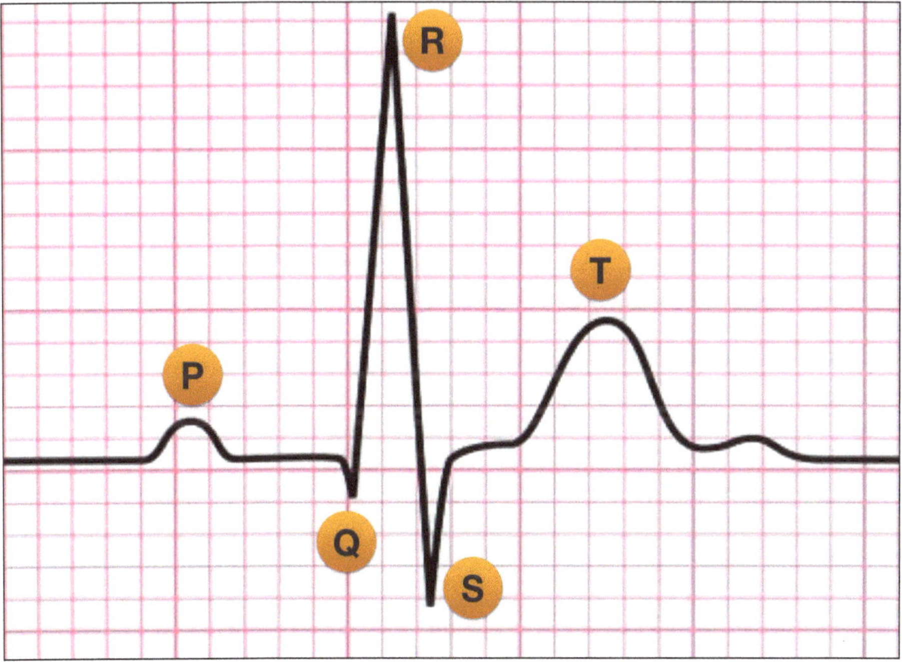

By analyzing the shape, size, and timing of these waves in each lead, we can gain valuable insights into the health and function of the heart.

SQUARES AND SECONDS

The foundation of an ECG recording is a gridded sheet featuring **squares of two sizes.**

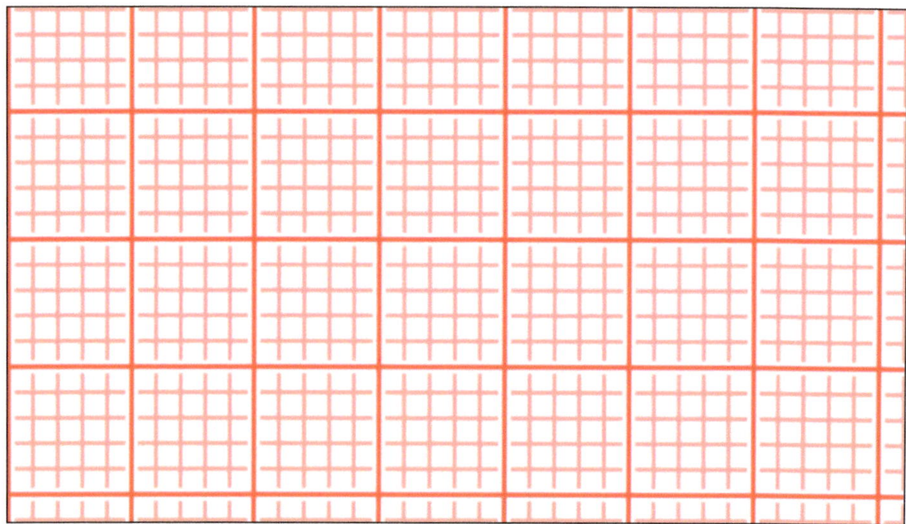

Each large square measure 5 millimeters and **represents 200 milliseconds** of the heart's electrical activity.

A standard ECG travels across the paper at a speed of **25 millimeters per second**, meaning each large square equates to 200 milliseconds.

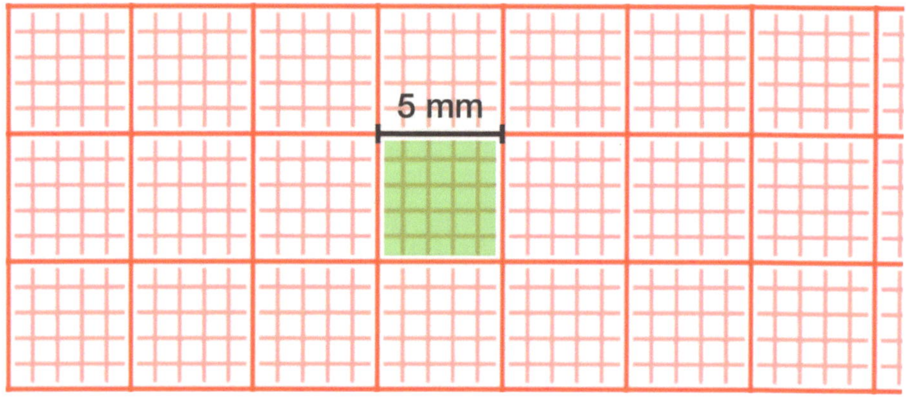

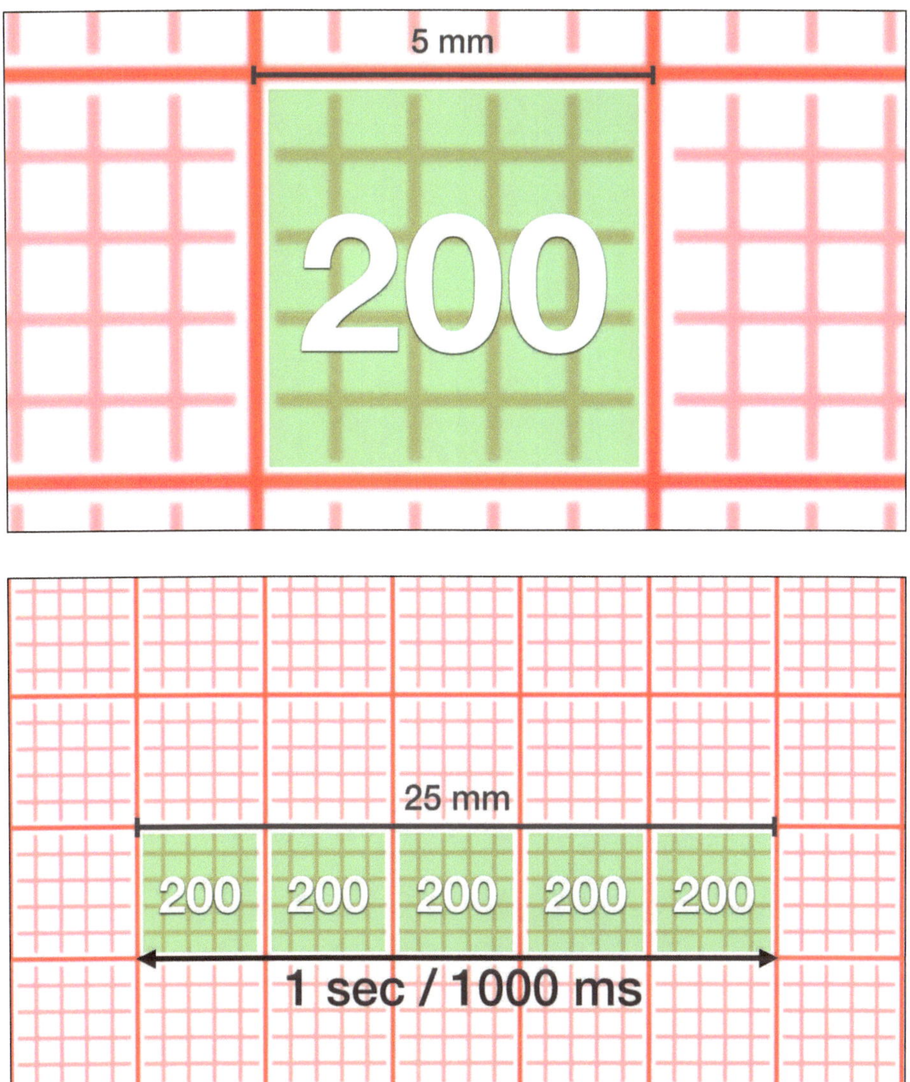

These **large squares are further divided into 5 smaller squares, each 1 millimeter long** and **representing 40 milliseconds.**

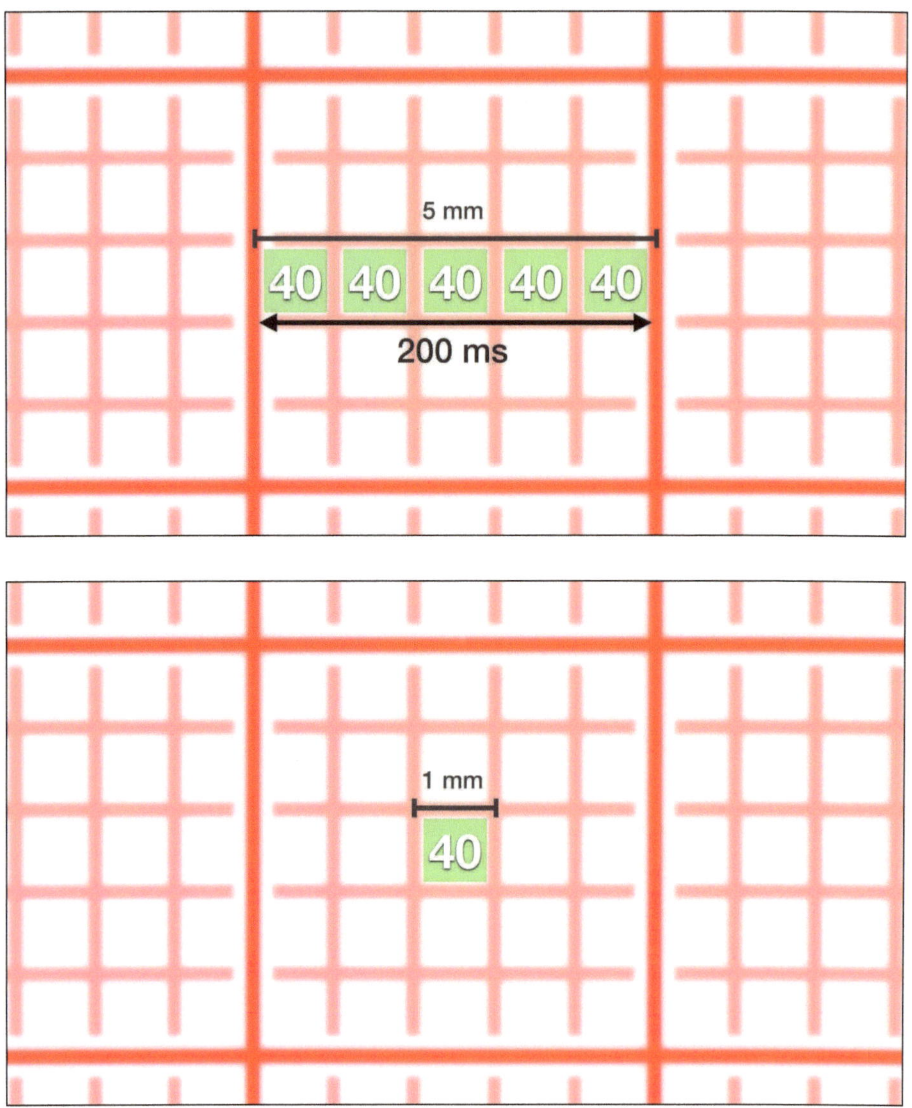

The **vertical axis** of the grid also uses a 5-millimeter scale. Here, **2 large squares (or 10 millimeters) correspond to 1 millivolt (mV)**.

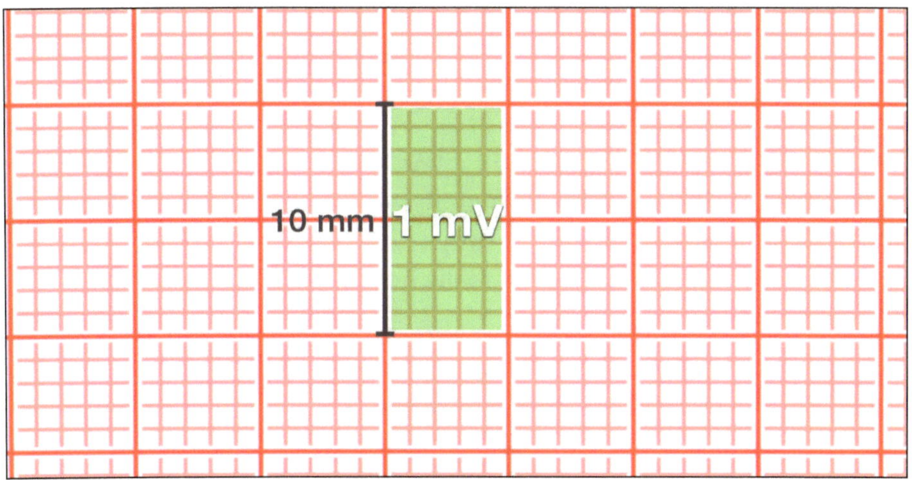

An ECG typically records the heart's activity for 10 seconds. This recording includes a continuous tracing of **lead II**, often called the **rhythm strip**, which provides a long-term view of the heart rhythm over the entire 10 seconds.

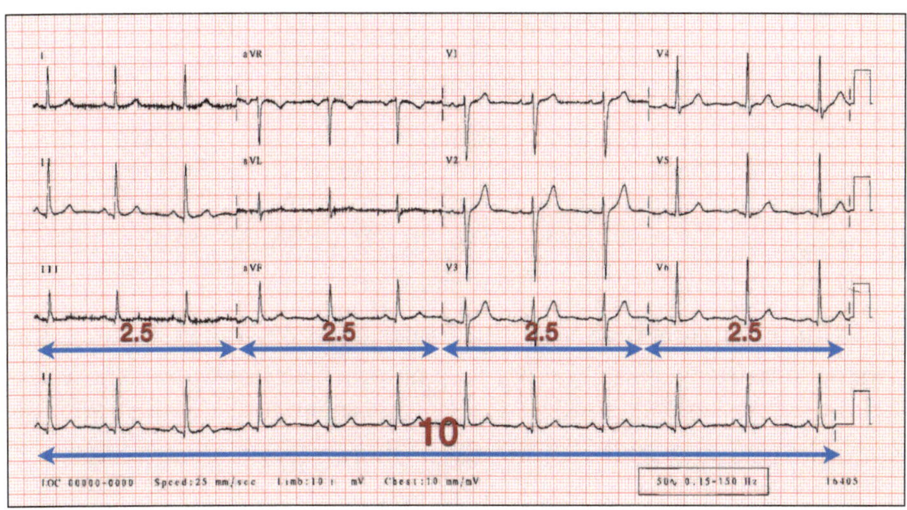

Additionally, multiple leads (often 12) are captured, each lasting 2.5 seconds. These leads capture the electrical activity from various angles of the heart, providing a more detailed picture for analysis.

Identification is the first step in ECG interpretation. While it may seem like a basic step, accurately identifying the patient is critical in ECG interpretation. Errors can occur when dealing with multiple patients, leading to misdiagnosis and potentially harmful consequences.

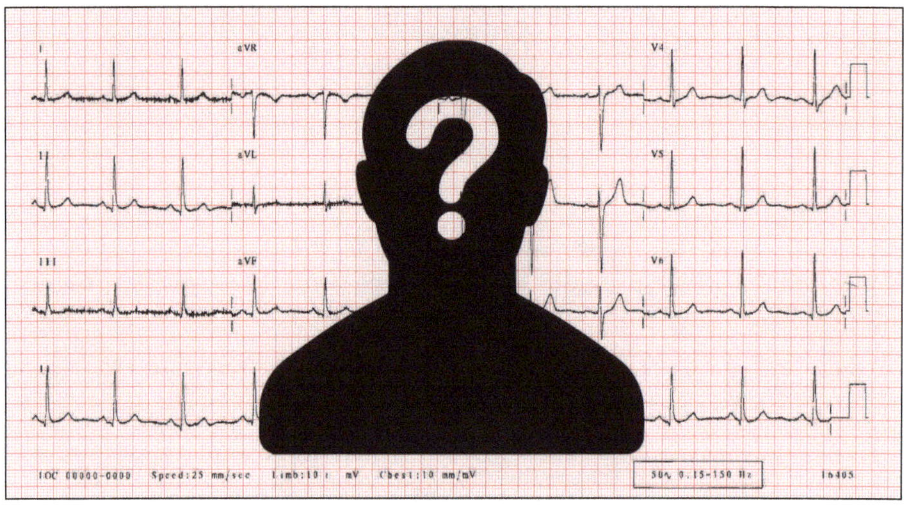

Verify patient identity by matching the name on the ECG **exactly** to the patient and **cross-referencing the ID** with their medical record. This prevents misinterpretation and ensures accurate diagnosis.

Clinical Context: Before ECG interpretation, understanding the patient's history is crucial. Look for symptoms like chest pain, dizziness, and any suspected diagnoses related to heart rhythm or function. This context guides your analysis towards the most relevant abnormalities.

VALIDITY

Validating an ECG is crucial for accurate analysis. Scrutinize **calibration** and **electrode placement** for any irregularities before interpretation.

STANDARD CALIBRATION: For reliable ECG analysis, ensure standard calibration settings (**25 mm/sec & 10 mm/1mV**) are met. This information is typically printed on the ECG itself. Additionally, a **calibration box**, often a square measuring **1 large square wide and 2 large squares tall**, is present at the beginning or end of the ECG leads. This box serves as a separate reference point for the actual recording settings.

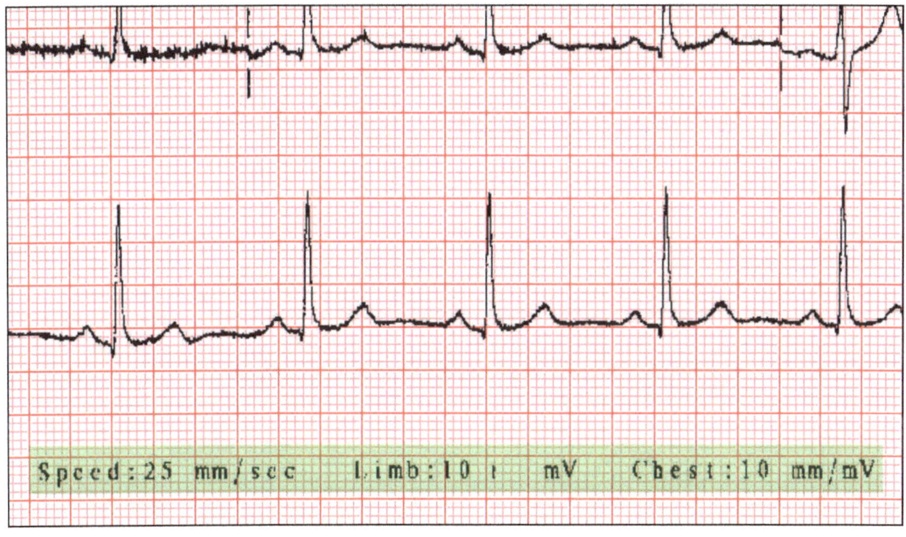

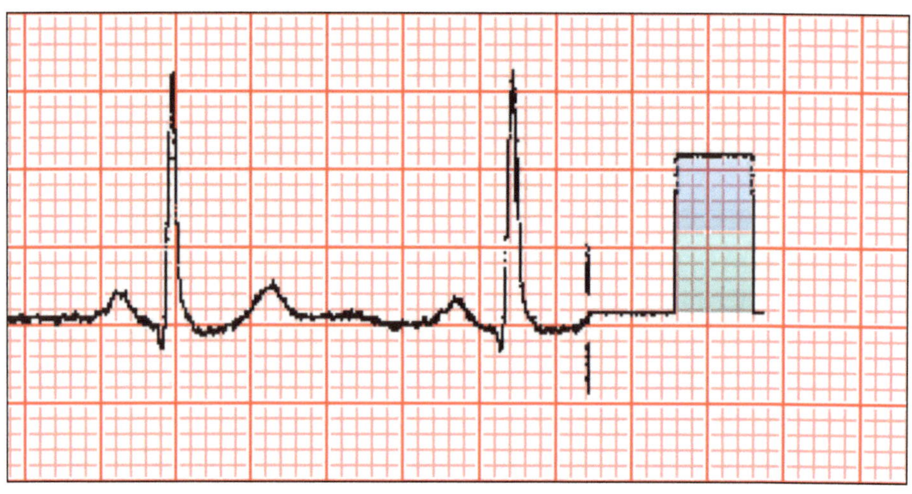

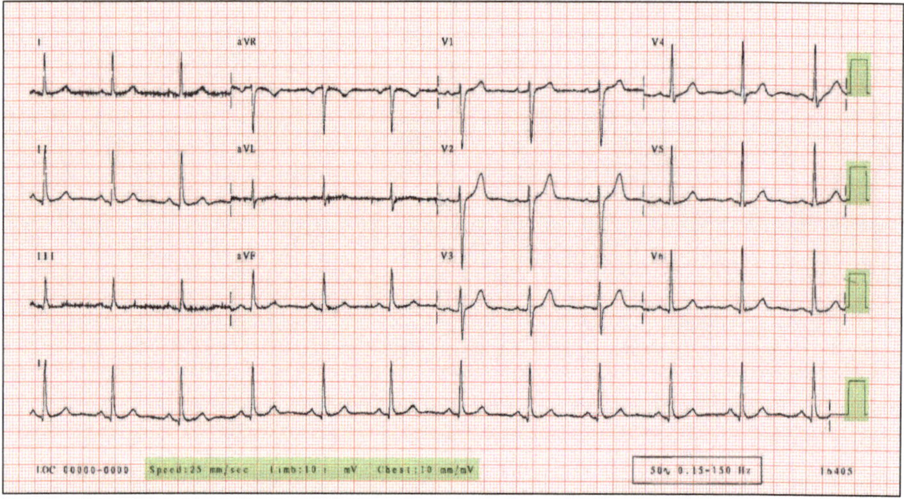

ELECTRODE PLACEMENT: It is quite frequent to mix up the electrodes while recording an ECG, specifically right arm and left arm electrodes. In such cases, the interpretation will be wrong as the tracing gets altered. Hence, it is necessary to recognise and correct it first.

Review leads I, II, and III for signs of incorrect limb electrode placement. This may include:

- **Inversion of all waves (P, QRS, and T)** in ANY of these leads.

- **A near-flat line** appearing in ANY of leads I, II, or III.

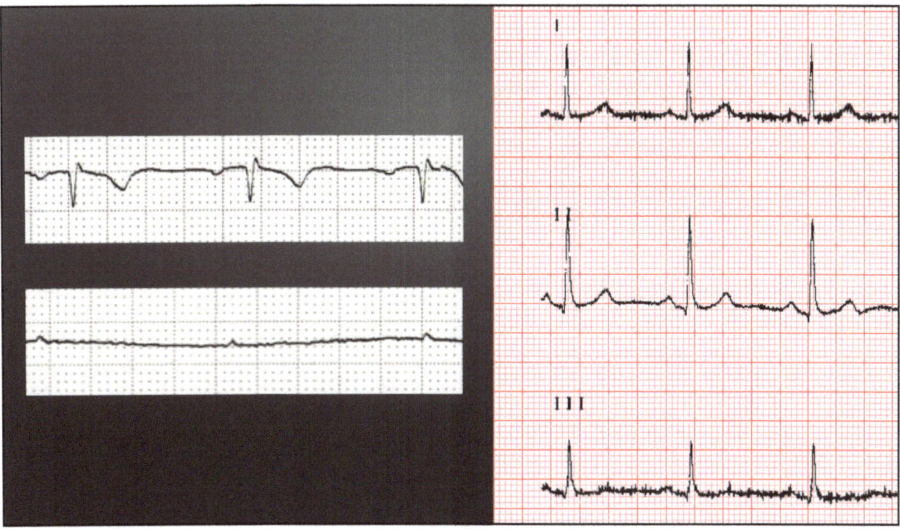

Following correction of electrode placement (right image), lead II inversions seen previously (left image) completely resolved.

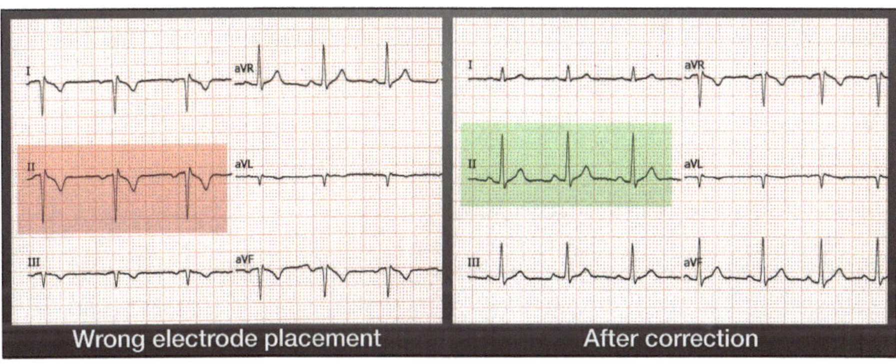

As seen in the next illustration, correcting electrode misplacement resulted in a significant normalization of the lead I tracing.

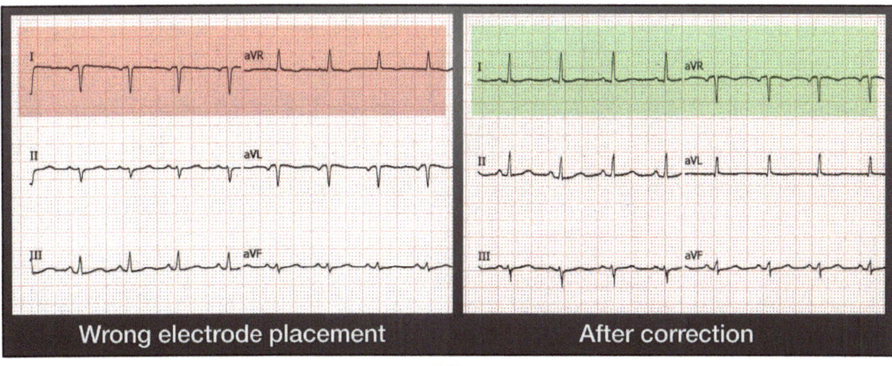

Lead aVR offers a valuable tool for detecting misplacement, as normally inverted waves become upright with incorrect right arm electrode placement. However, as illustrated in the next illustration, reversed left arm and leg electrodes can maintain inverted aVR waves, masking the wrong electrode placement.

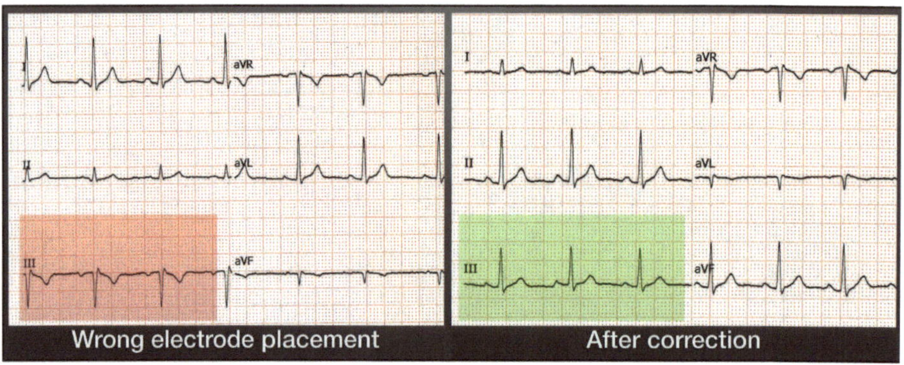

The next illustration further emphasizes the impact of electrode placement. Note the reappearance of all waves in lead III (right image) after correction, compared to the initial flat line (left image).

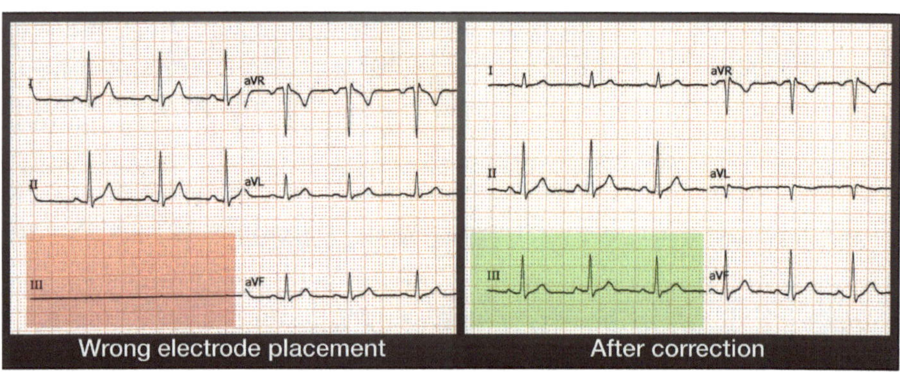

In the chest leads, as illustrated on the next page, **normal R wave progression** shows **a gradual increase in upright deflection from V1 to V6.** Conversely, the **abnormal R wave progression** can be caused by factors like **incorrect chest electrode placement.**

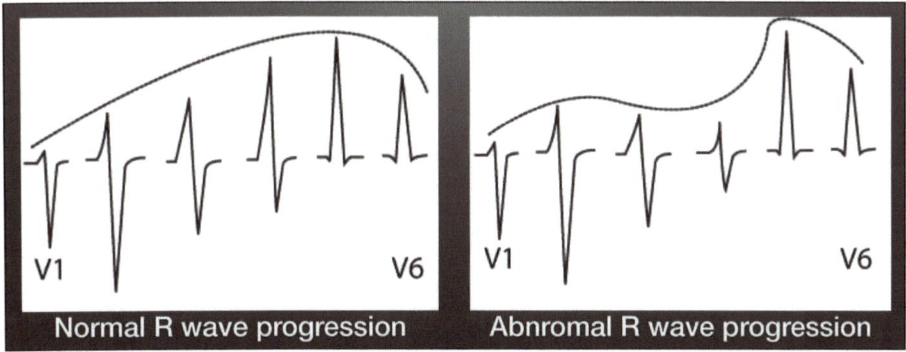

Normal R wave progression | Abnromal R wave progression

The next illustration provides a clear picture of the problem. The reversed V1 and V3 electrodes on the right image resulted in the abnormal R wave progression discussed earlier. The corrected placement on the left image shows the normal R wave progression once again.

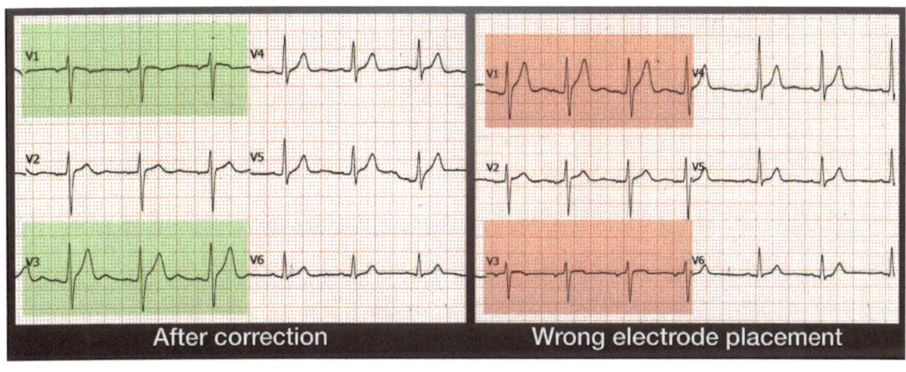

After correction | Wrong electrode placement

RATE

The heart rate can be calculated by looking at the rhythm strip (lead II) on ECG.

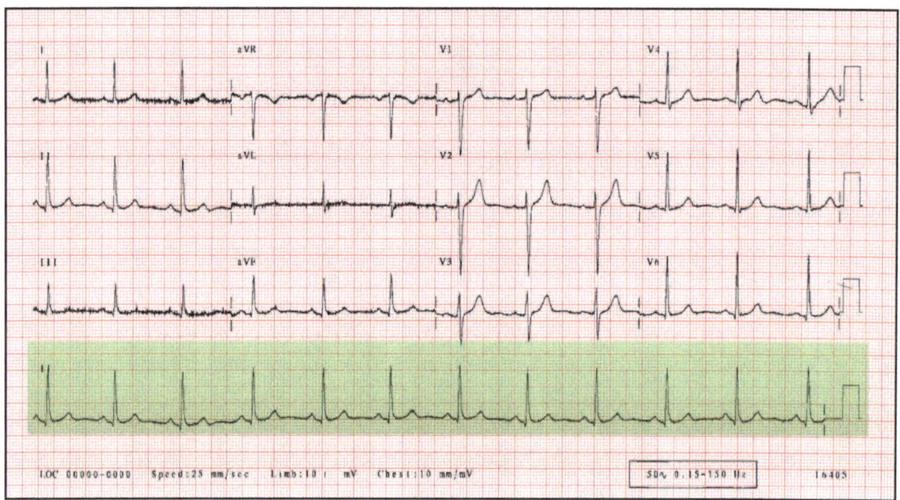

Count all the QRS complexes on a 10-second ECG rhythm strip. Multiply that number by 6. This gives you the approximate heart rate in beats per minute (bpm) because 10 seconds x 6 = 60 seconds (1 minute).

This method works well for both regular and irregular rhythms.

Example:

There are a total of 12 QRS complexes in this rhythm strip. 12 multiplied by 6 is equal to 72 is the approximate heart rate in this case.

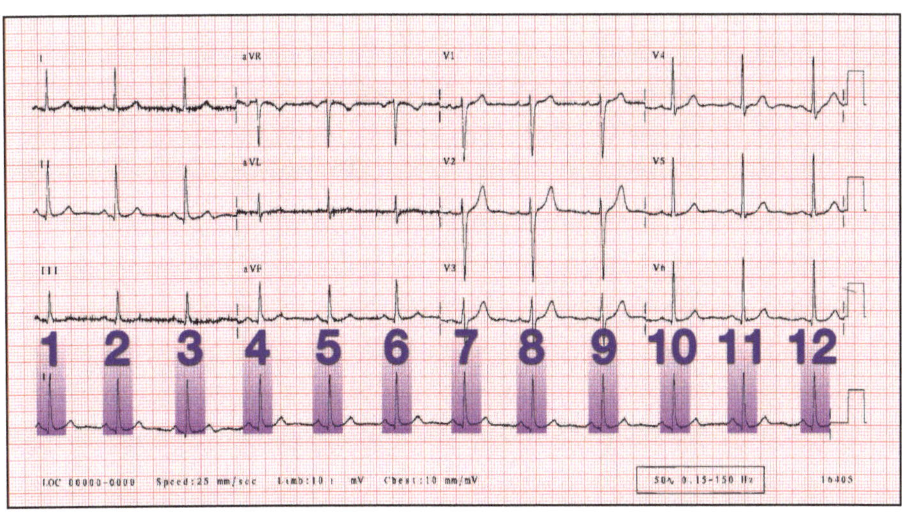

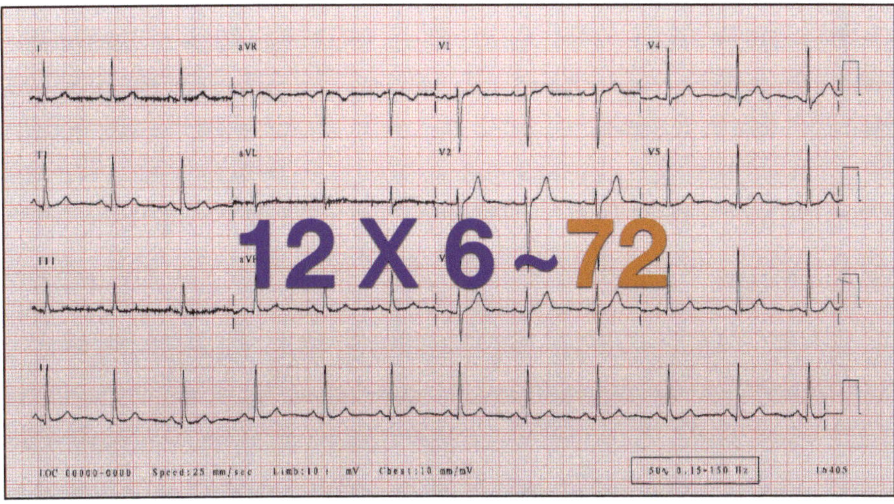

Here's an **alternative method**:

Identify two consecutive QRS complexes. (*Tip: Choose a QRS complex which coincides with the starting of a large square*). **Count the large squares between** those **two QRS complexes**.

Divide 300 by the number of large squares counted. This will give you the approximate heart rate in bpm.

Limitation: This second method is not accurate for irregular rhythms because the space between QRS complexes will vary.

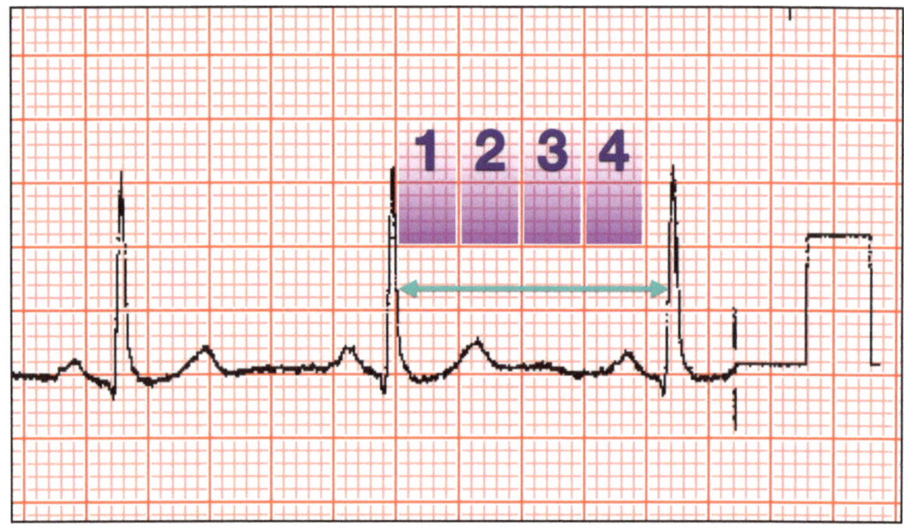

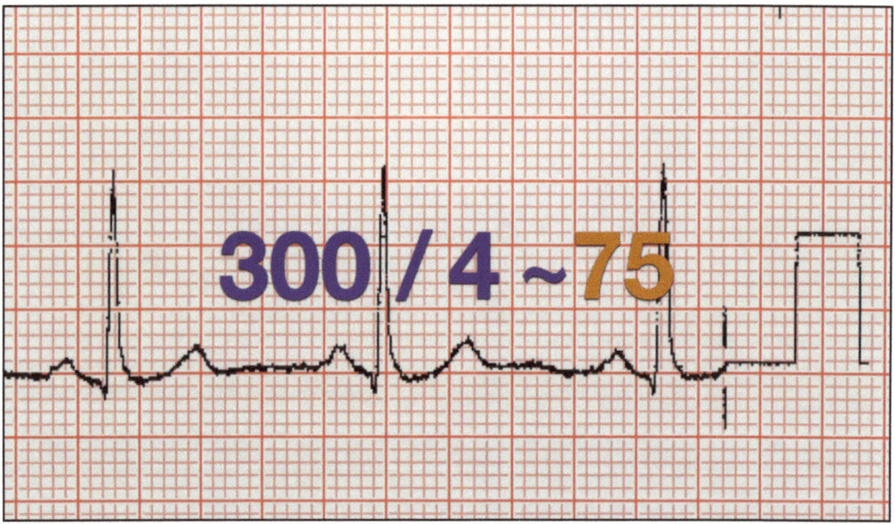

A **normal heart rate** (between 60 and 100 bpm) typically translates to a distance of **3 to 5 large squares between consecutive QRS complexes** (RR interval). If the distance is **less than 3 large squares**, it suggests a heart rate exceeding 100 bpm, which is called **tachycardia**. Conversely, a distance **greater than 5 large squares** between QRS complexes might indicate a heart rate slower than 60 bpm, known as **bradycardia**.

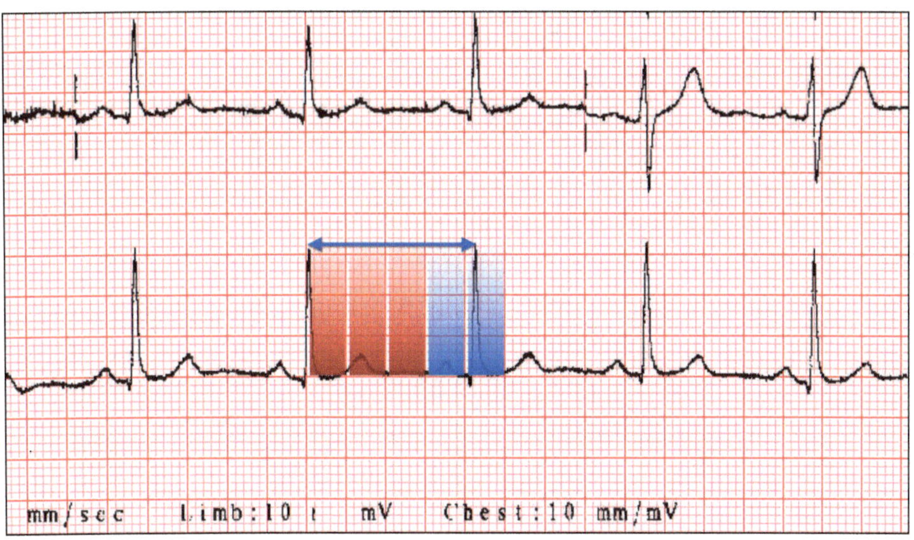

mm/sec   Limb:10   mV   Chest:10 mm/mV

RHYTHM

For a quick and efficient assessment of heart rhythm, focus on the rhythm strip (lead II) on the 12-lead ECG. This provides a clear picture of the electrical activity.

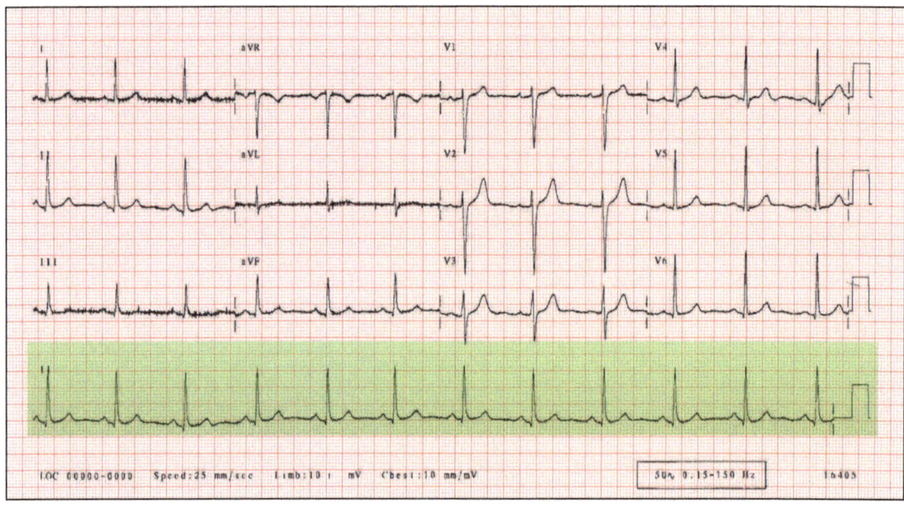

Let's begin by analyzing a normal ECG rhythm and explore the essential steps involved in rhythm analysis.

Normal Sinus Rhythm

The very first step in analyzing ECG rhythm is to assess the regularity of the QRS complexes. This is achieved by measuring the intervals between consecutive QRS complexes. **Consistent spacing** between these peaks tells us we're dealing with a **regular rhythm**, while **any variation in spacing indicates** an **irregular rhythm**.

To assess regularity visually, a simple technique can be employed. Place a piece of paper on the rhythm strip and mark the peaks of the QRS complexes. Slide the paper one QRS complex at a time and observe if the subsequent QRS peaks align with the previously marked lines. Consistent alignment indicates a regular rhythm, while deviations suggest irregularity.

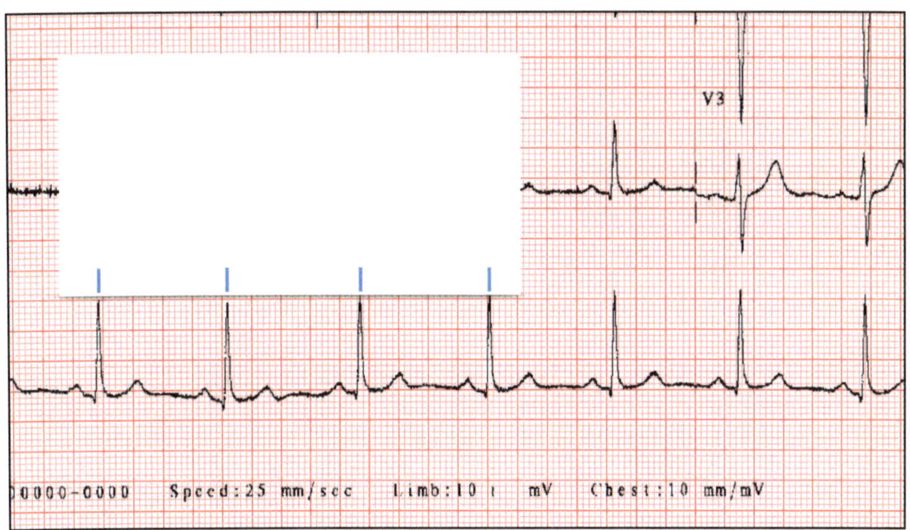

V3
00000-0000   Speed:25 mm/sec   Limb:10 t   mV   Chest:10 mm/mV

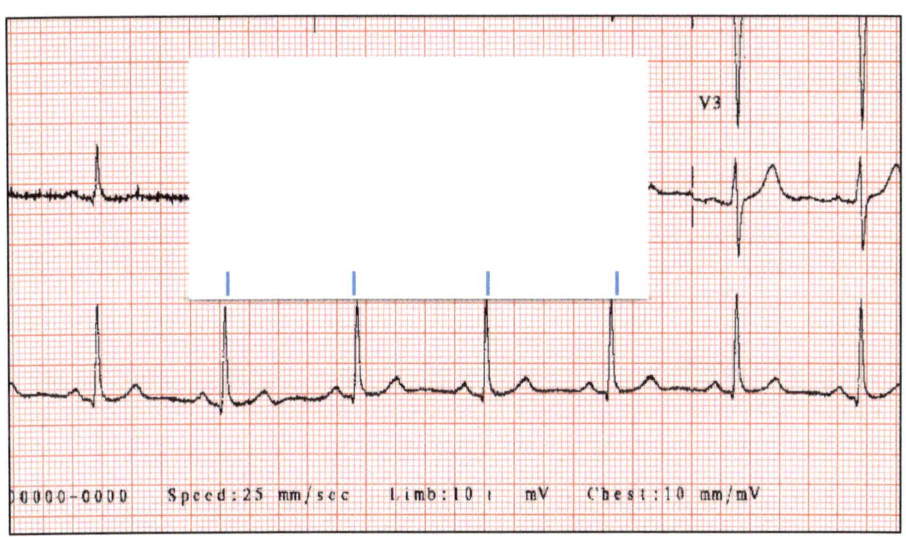

V3
00000-0000   Speed:25 mm/sec   Limb:10 t   mV   Chest:10 mm/mV

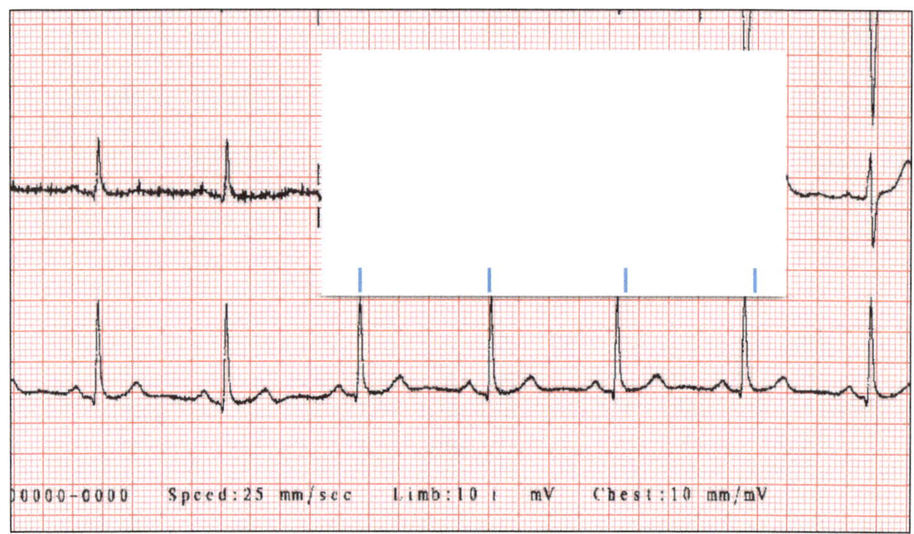

The second step is to determine whether the **QRS complex is wide or narrow**.

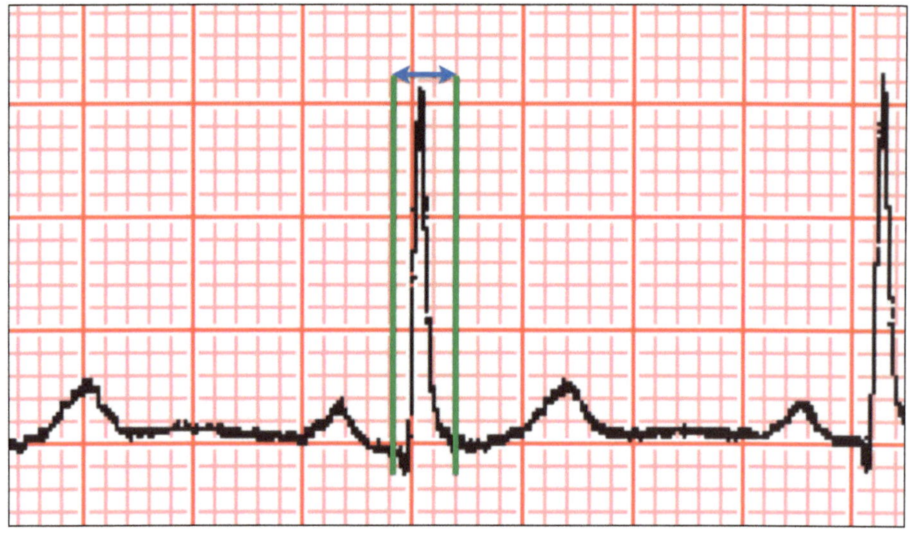

The QRS complex, reflecting the electrical activity in the lower heart chambers (ventricles), is measured from its initial deflection (Q wave) to the end of the S wave. A **narrow QRS** (normal) is usually **less than 3 small squares wide**. A **wide QRS** (may indicate an issue) is **3 small squares wide or more**.

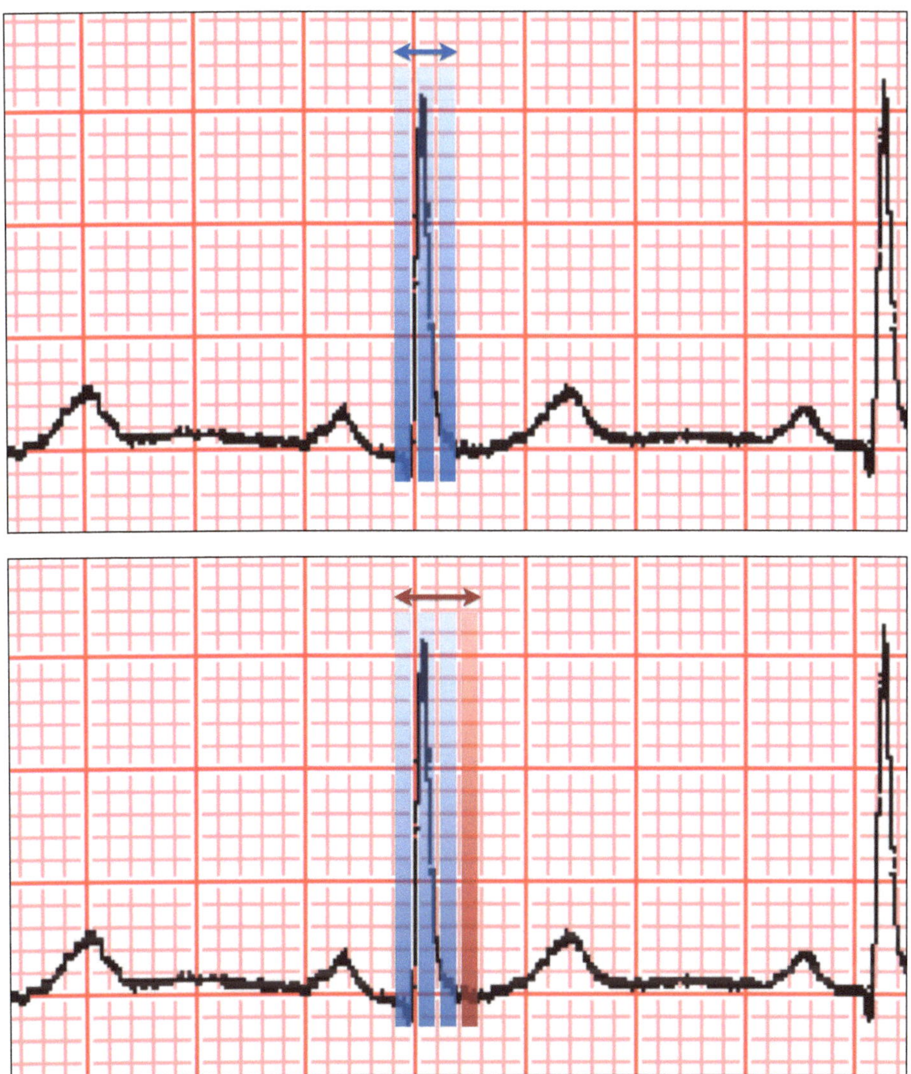

The third step focuses on the **relationship between the P waves and QRS complexes**. These electrical signals reveal how impulses travel through the heart. A **sinus rhythm**, shows a consistent pattern: each **P wave** is followed by a **QRS complex** and each **QRS complex** is preceded by a **P wave**.

Some rhythms, such as **sinus tachycardia (rate over 100 bpm)** and **sinus bradycardia (rate under 60 bpm)**, follow this sinus pattern and are generally **physiological**.

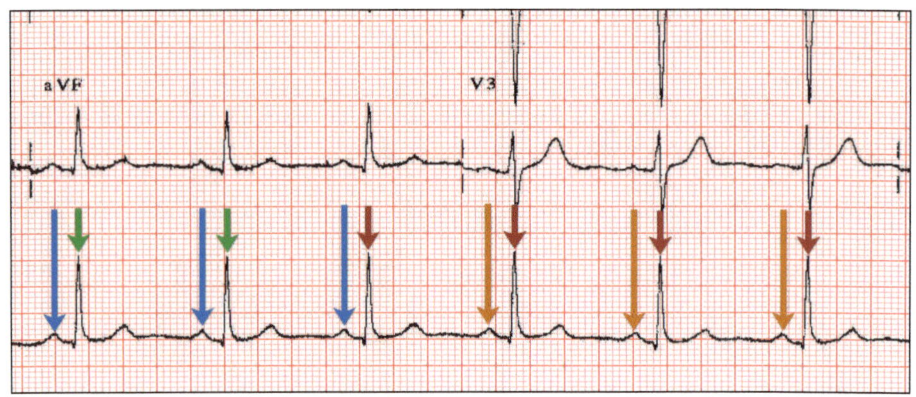

Beyond the Normal Beat:
Exploring Tachyarrhythmia (fast rhythms)

To identify tachyarrhythmias (rate over 100 bpm), the ECG shows an interval of **less than 3 large squares between QRS consecutive complexes.**

Atrial Flutter

Step 1: Check Rhythm Regularity

Look at the QRS complexes on the ECG. This consistent spacing indicates a *regular* rhythm.

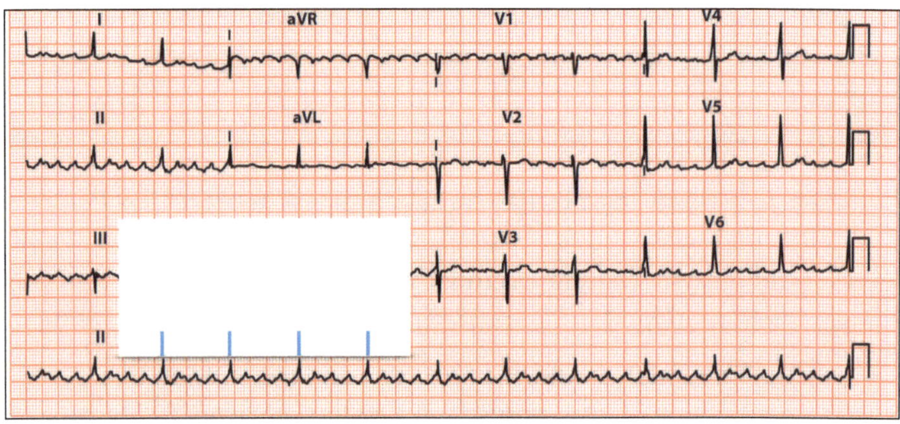

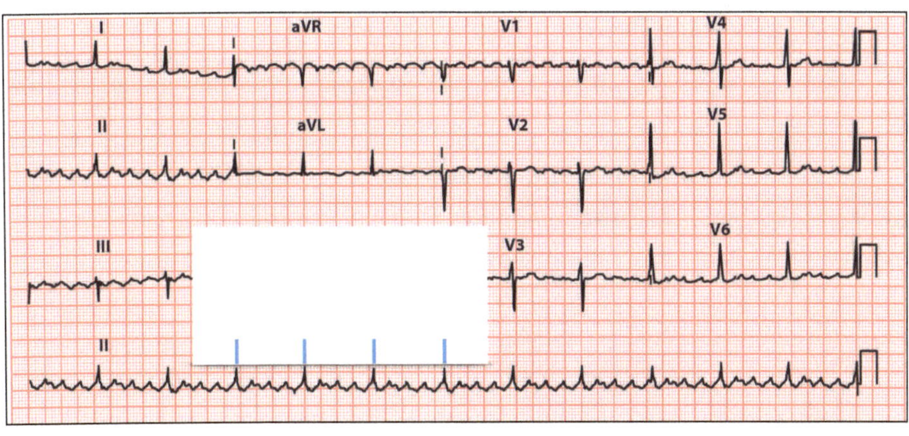

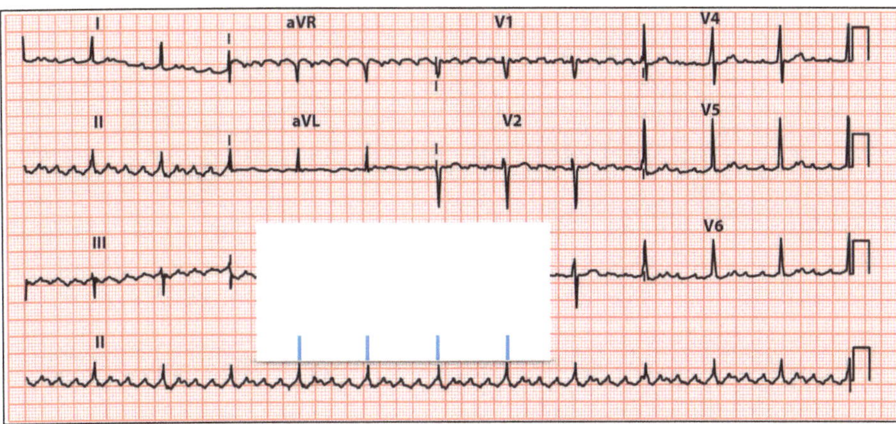

Step 2: QRS Width

Next, let's look at the width of the QRS complex. In this case, the QRS complex is ***narrow***.

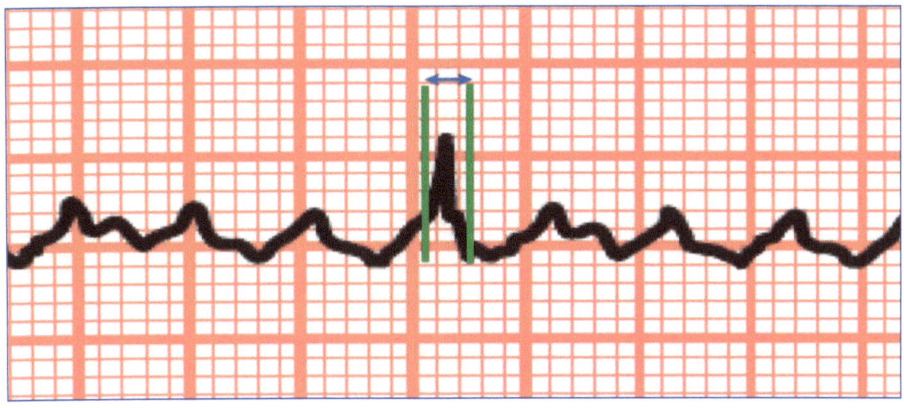

Step 3: P Wave and QRS Complex Relationship

Look at the ECG. Here, you see *multiple P waves* that are not followed by a QRS complex, indicating an abnormal P:QRS ratio.

*"In **atrial flutter**, the relationship between P and QRS waves resembles a woman named 'QRS' who is committed to her boyfriend 'P' (representing **regular** QRS complexes), yet also involved with two other 'Ps' (symbolizing **flutter waves**)."*

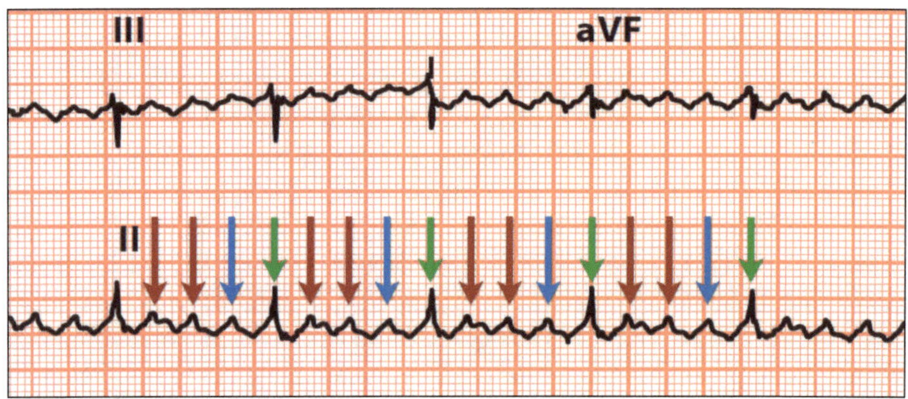

When the tips of the QRS complexes are covered, the baseline will appear wavy, giving a typical **saw-tooth appearance, which is one of the characteristics of atrial flutter**.

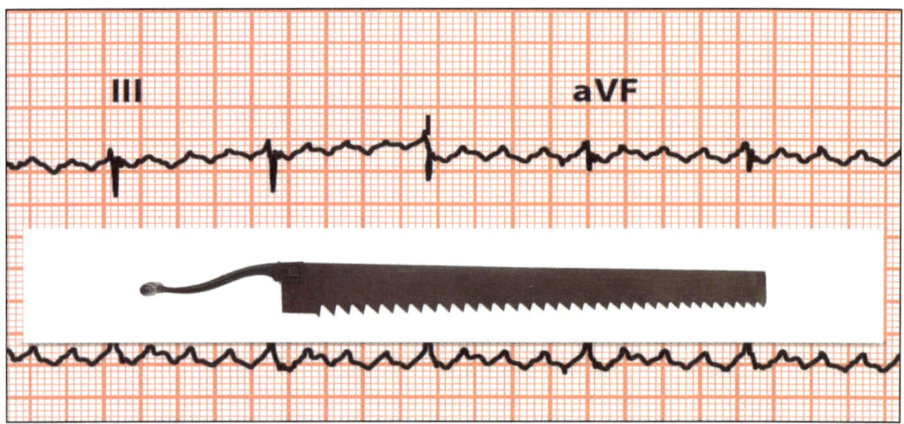

*"Tip: Follow 'R' - 'Q' - 'P' pneumonic when assessing a rhythm with tachy (fast) rate. Example: Rhythm: Regular, **QRS**: Narrow, **P**- waves: Multiple = Atrial Flutter."*

Supraventricular Tachycardia (SVT)

Step 1: Check Rhythm *'R'*egularity

Since the distance between each QRS complex is consistent, this rhythm is ***regular***.

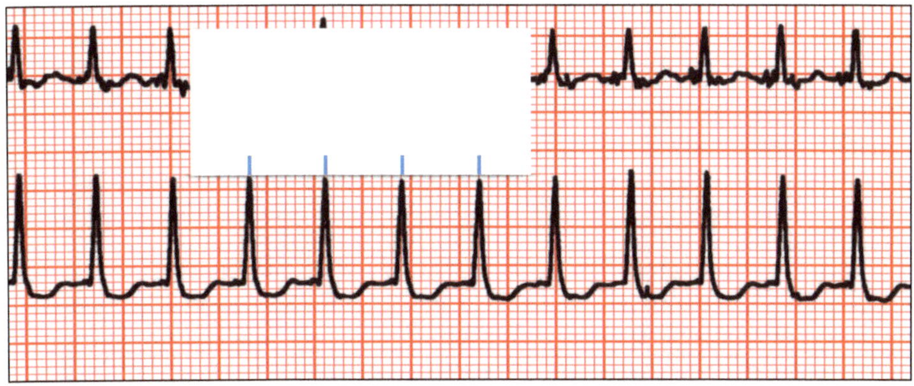

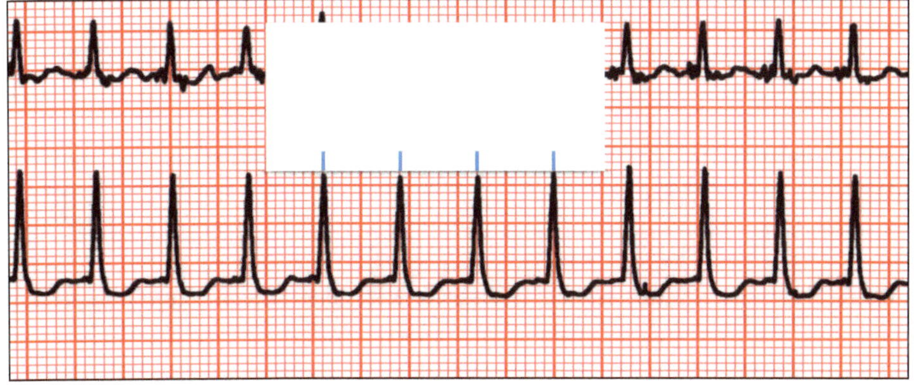

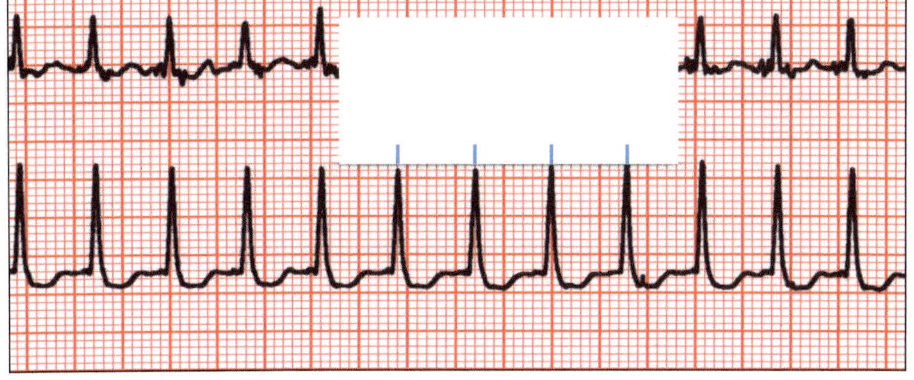

Step 2: 'Q'RS Width

Since the width of the QRS complex is less than 3 small squares on the ECG, it is considered a ***narrow*** QRS complex.

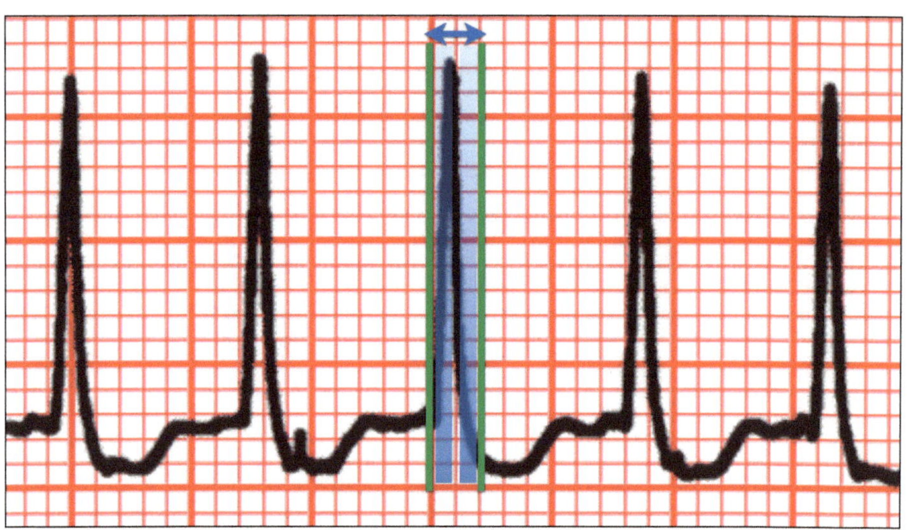

Step 3: 'P' Wave and QRS Complex Relationship

This rhythm shows clear **QRS complexes**, but there are ***no P waves*** before them.

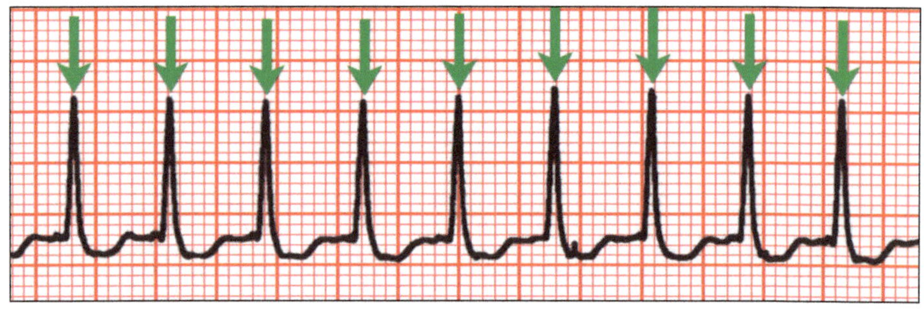

"Imagine **'QRS'** *as a single and **regular** lady named 'Sweety' (**SVT**). Unlike the girl with a boyfriend ('P' wave in atrial flutter), Sweety is consistently single, which means there are* **no preceding 'P' waves** *in her case."*

Rhythm: *Regular,* ***QRS:*** *Narrow and* ***P*** *waves: Absent = Supraventricular Tachycardia (SVT)*

Ventricular Tachycardia (VT)

Step 1: Check Rhythm *'R'*egularity

The distance between each QRS complex is consistent, suggesting a *regular* heart rhythm.

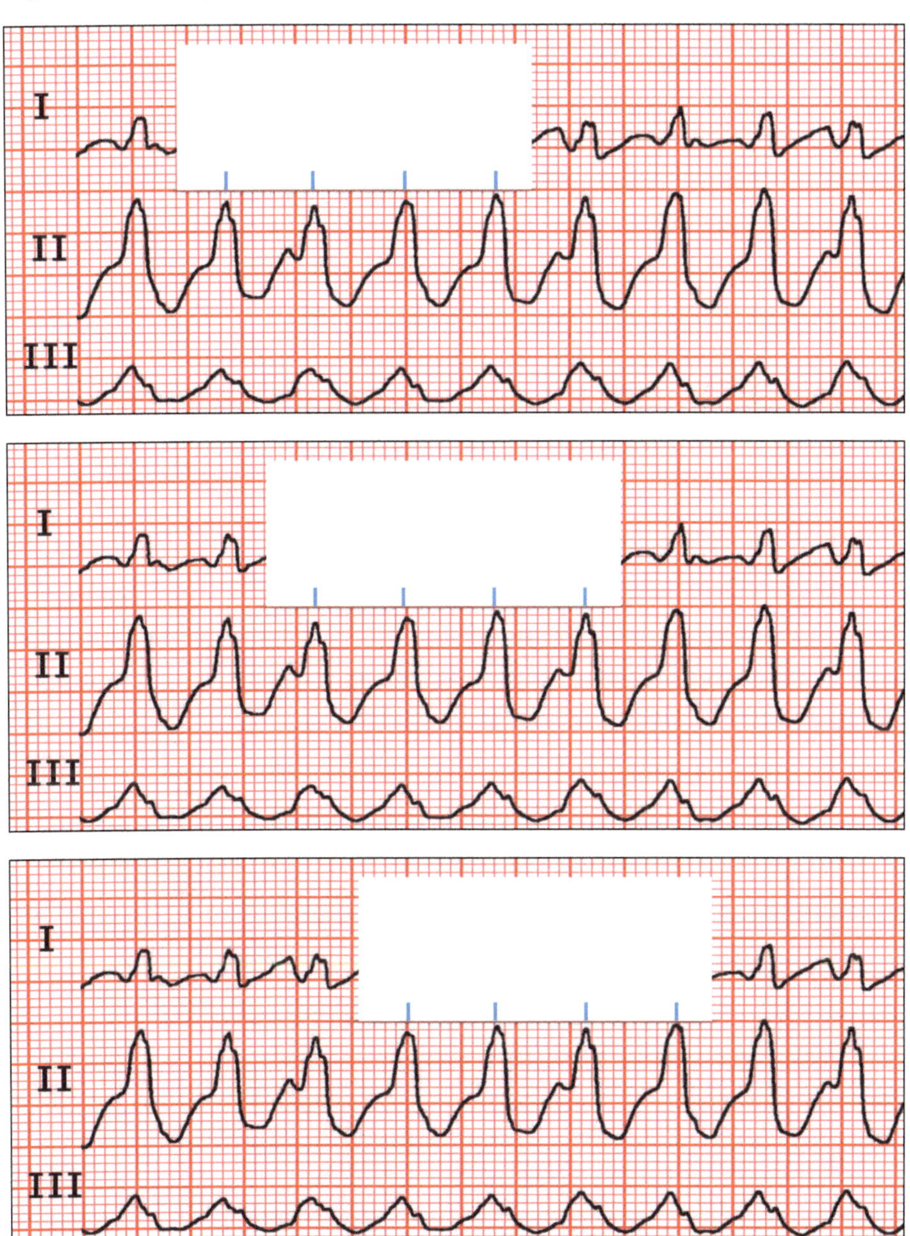

Step 2: 'Q'RS Width

The QRS complex measures greater than 3 small squares, indicating a *wide* QRS complex

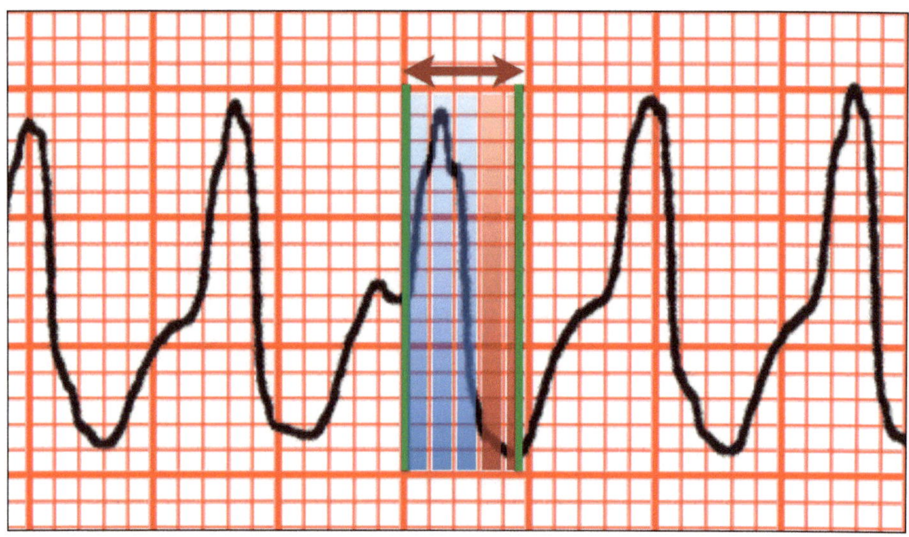

Step 3: 'P' Wave and QRS Complex Relationship

There are **no P waves** before the QRS complexes. (In some cases, tiny P waves might seem to blend with the QRS complexes. These are called dissociated P waves, but we'll disregard them for now to keep things straightforward).

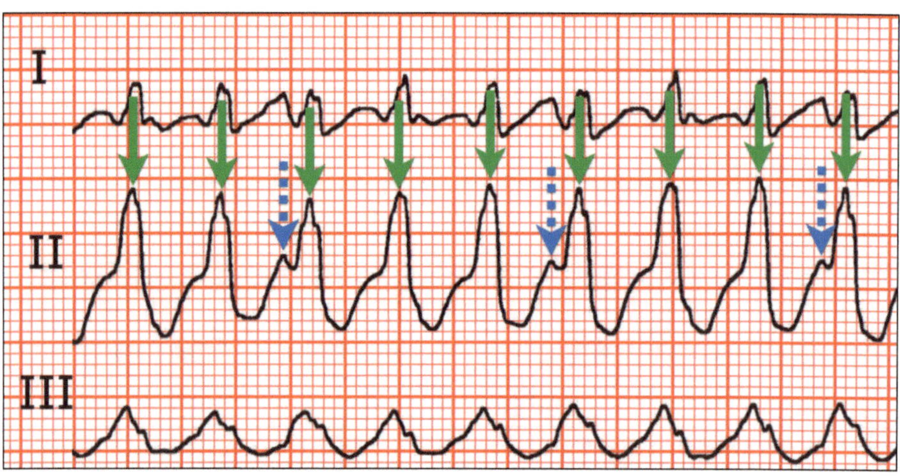

*"Imagine Sweety (SVT), a girl who resisted peer pressure to enter a relationship, maintaining her **regular rhythm**. However, the pressure eventually causes her frustration to grow, **widen**ing her 'QRS'. Sweety, no longer sweet, transforms into **VT (Ventricular Tachycardia)**."*

Rhythm: Regular, **Q**RS: Wide and **P** waves: Absent = Ventricular Tachycardia (VT)

Atrial Fibrillation

Step 1: Check Rhythm '**R**'egularity

In this rhythm strip, a crucial finding is that the QRS complexes, unlike those in previous examples, are not evenly spaced. They don't line up with the markings we've made on the paper, displaying irregular intervals between each complex. This inconsistency in spacing is a key indicator of an **irregular** heart rhythm.

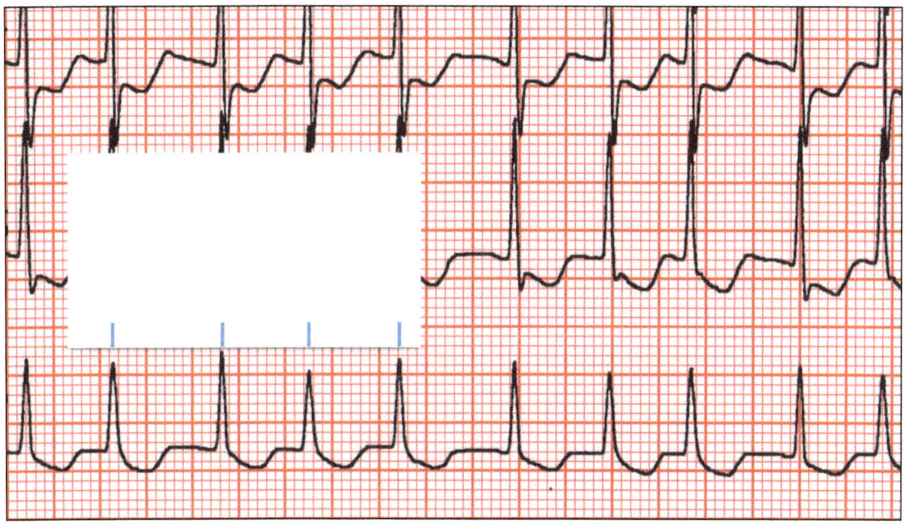

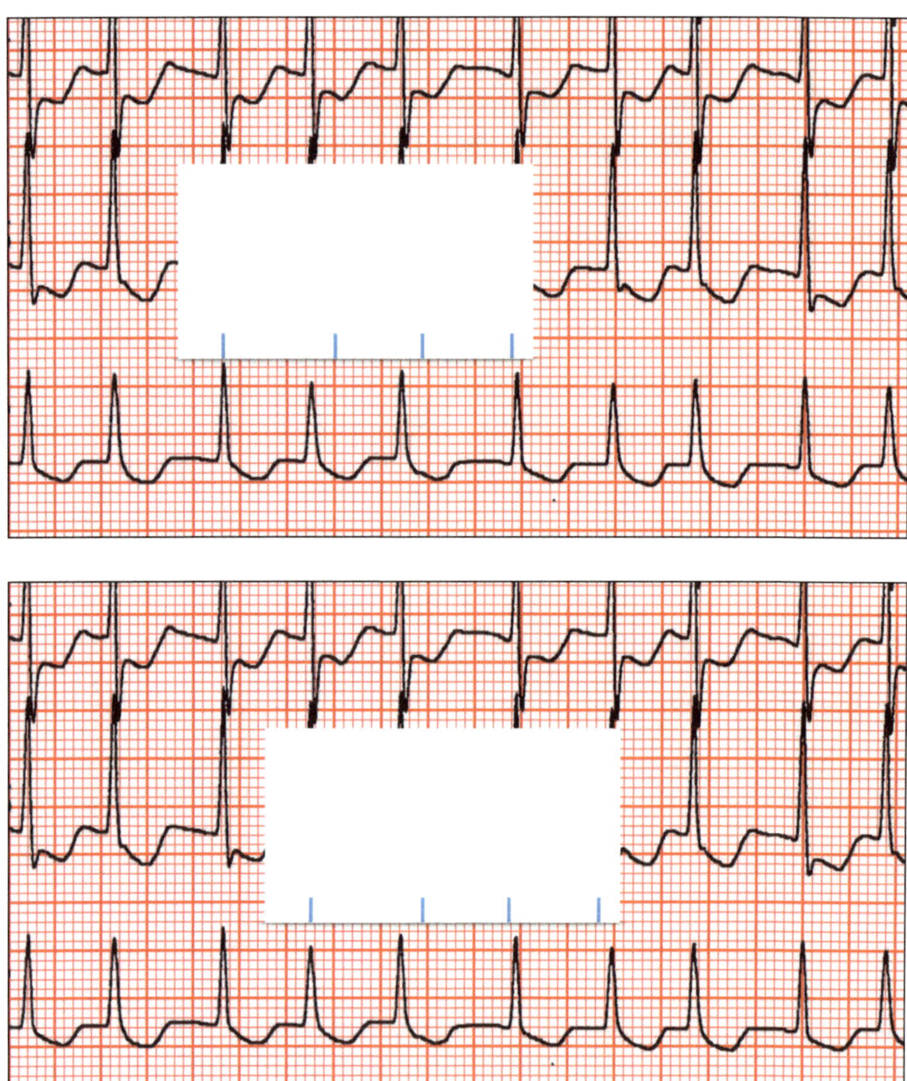

Step 2: 'Q'RS Width

The QRS complexes in this rhythm strip appear narrow, measuring less than 3 small squares on the ECG paper.

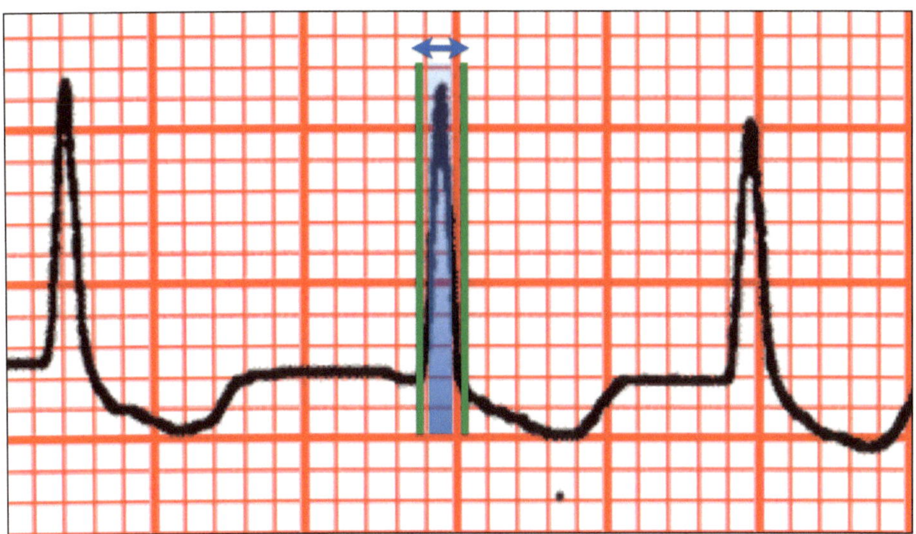

Step 3: 'P' Wave and QRS Complex Relationship

A strong indicator of this rhythm is the ***absence of P waves***.

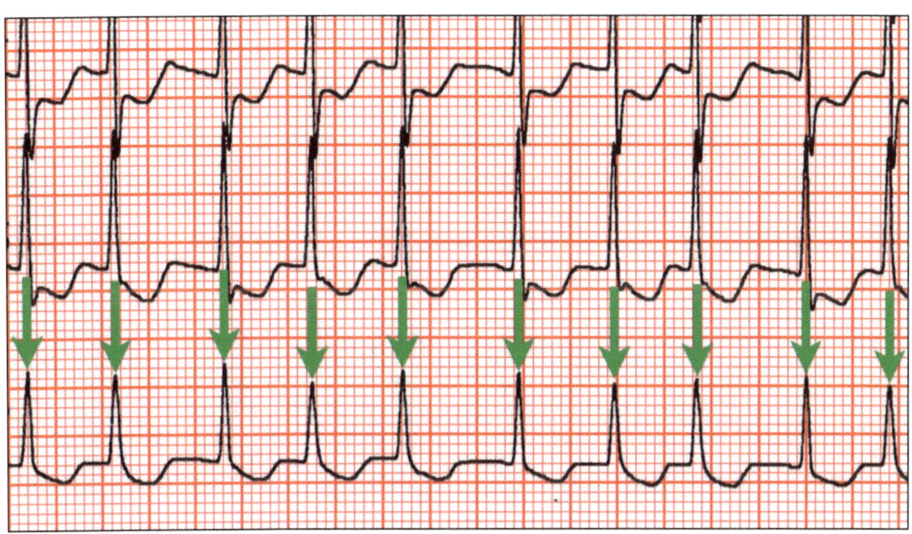

*"The boyfriends of the girl in atrial flutter discover her affairs with other guys and leave her. Devastated by their departure, she becomes emotionally **irregular**, marked by the absence of steady relationships (no P waves). This transformation leads her to become **atrial fibrillation**."*

*Rhythm: Irregular, **QRS**: Narrow and **P** waves: Absent = Atrial Fibrillation*

Polymorphic Ventricular Tachycardia (PVT)

Torsades de Pointes, a type of **Polymorphic VT**, differs from regular VT by its ***irregular*** and twisting ECG pattern, complicating clinical management and treatment.

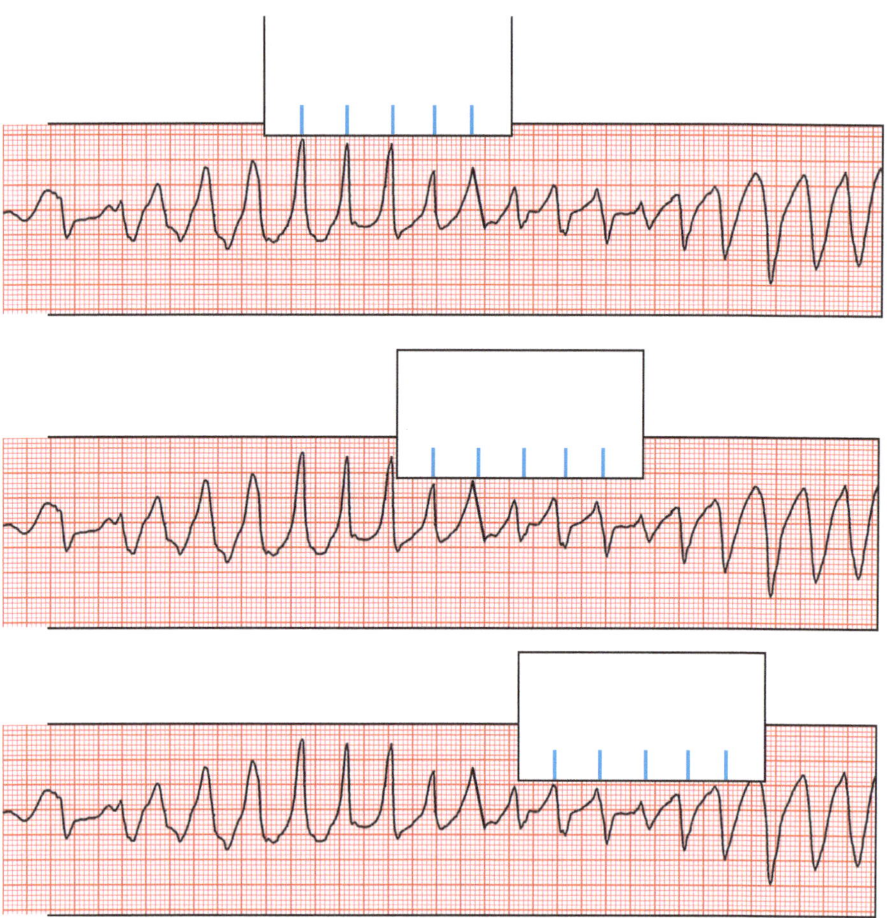

Similar to VT, Torsades de Pointes also exhibits ***wide QRS complexes*** and ***lacks identifiable P waves*** on the ECG.

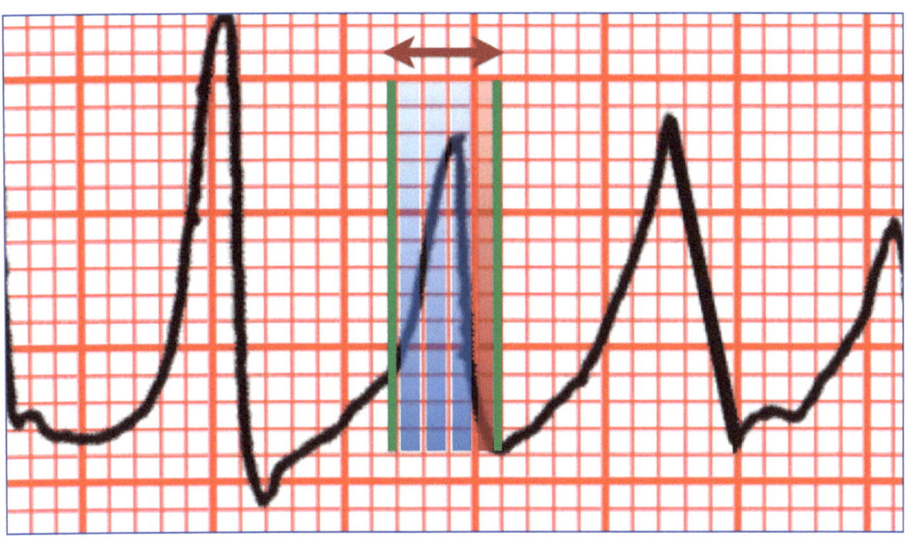

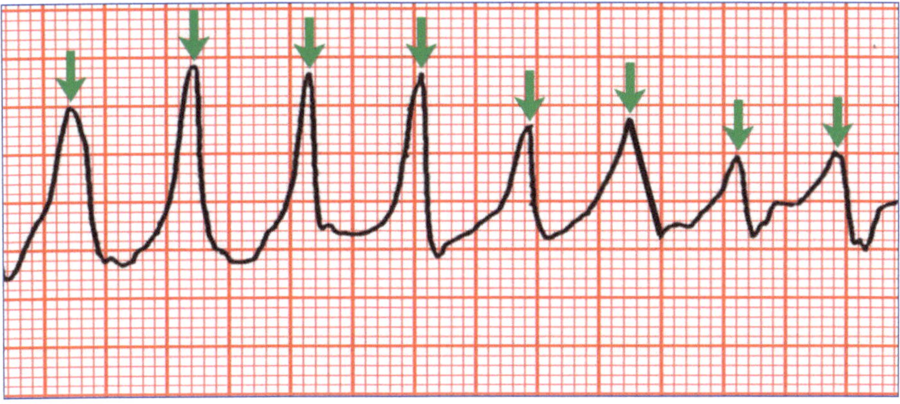

*"Put simply, **when ventricular tachycardia (VT) becomes irregular, it transforms into polymorphic VT,** with Torsades de Pointes being a specific subtype of this irregular rhythm."*

R*hythm: Irregular,* **Q***RS: Wide and* **P** *waves: Absent = Polymorphic Ventricular Tachycardia (PVT).*

Ventricular Fibrillation

Ventricular fibrillation (VF) is a life-threatening arrhythmia with a **chaotic, irregular pattern** and **no defined waveforms**. It should be quickly recognized on the monitor and treated immediately with defibrillation (DC shock) and CPR as **the patient is pulseless and in cardiac arrest**. In such emergencies, obtaining a formal ECG is neither necessary, nor practical.

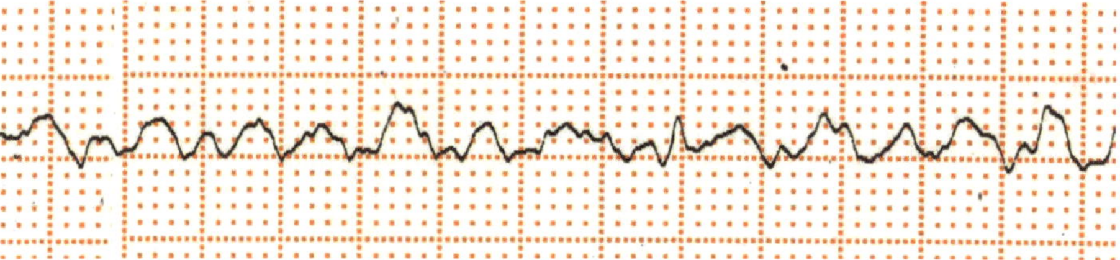

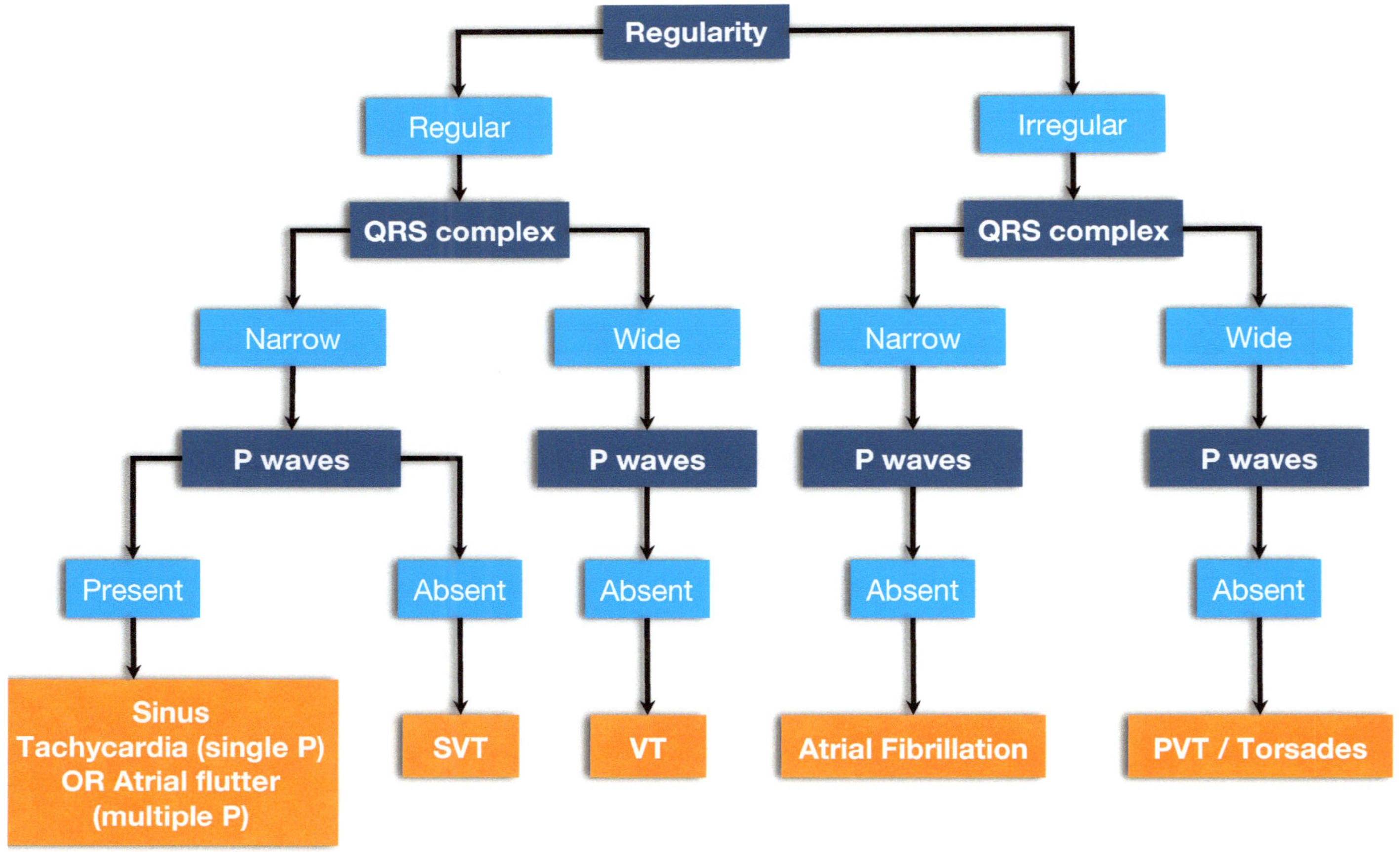

Regularity
Regular
Irregular
QRS complex
QRS complex
Narrow
Wide
Narrow
Wide
P waves
P waves
P waves
P waves
Present
Absent
Absent
Absent
Absent
Sinus Tachycardia (single P) OR Atrial flutter (multiple P)
SVT
VT
Atrial Fibrillation
PVT / Torsades

The Slower Side of Rhythm:
Understanding Bradyarrhythmia (slow rhythms)

Now, shifting to bradyarrhythmias, these rhythms, characterized by a rate of less than 60 bpm, are identified on the ECG by an interval of **more than 5 large squares between consecutive QRS complexes**.

Sinus Bradycardia

Step 1: Check Rhythm **'R'**egularity

Since the QRS complexes align precisely with the markings on the paper, their spacing is consistent and equidistant, indicating that this rhythm is *regular* in nature.

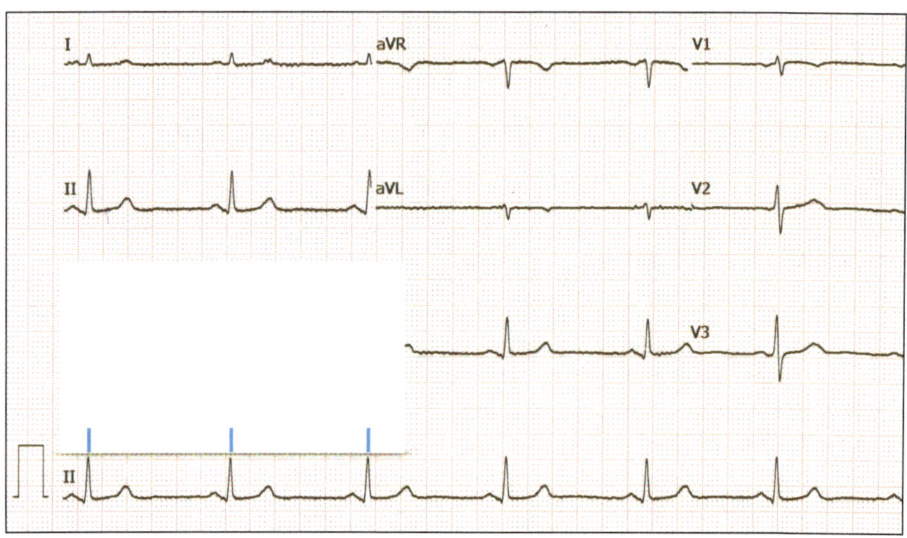

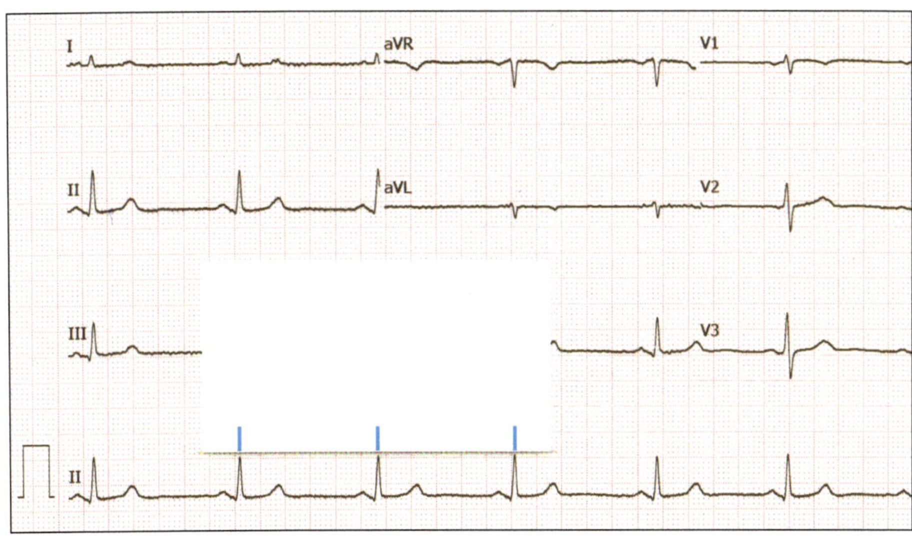

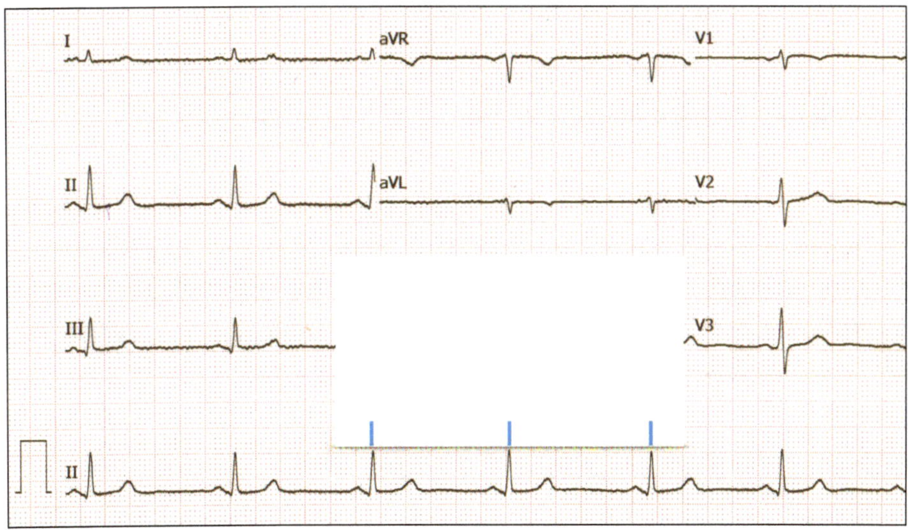

Step 2: 'Q'RS Width

The QRS complex appears **_narrow_** in this rhythm, measuring less than 3 small squares on the ECG.

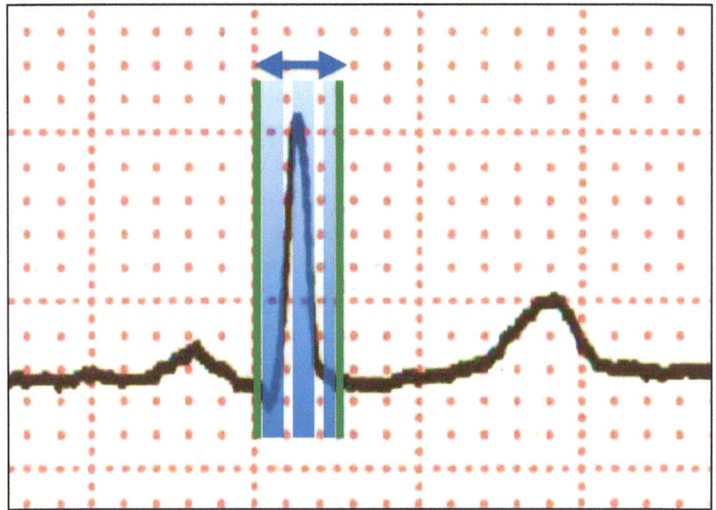

Up to this point, the first two steps in rhythm interpretation remain consistent whether assessing fast (tachy) or slow (brady) rhythms. However, there's a slight adjustment in step three for slow rhythms, where we focus on the time interval between the P wave and the QRS complex, requiring an understanding of what constitutes the PR interval.

The **PR interval** is measured from the **beginning of the P wave to the onset of the QRS complex** on an ECG. Typically, **a normal PR interval ranges between 3 to 5 small squares. If the PR interval extends beyond 5 small squares, it is considered prolonged**, indicating potential delays in the electrical conduction between the atria and the ventricles.

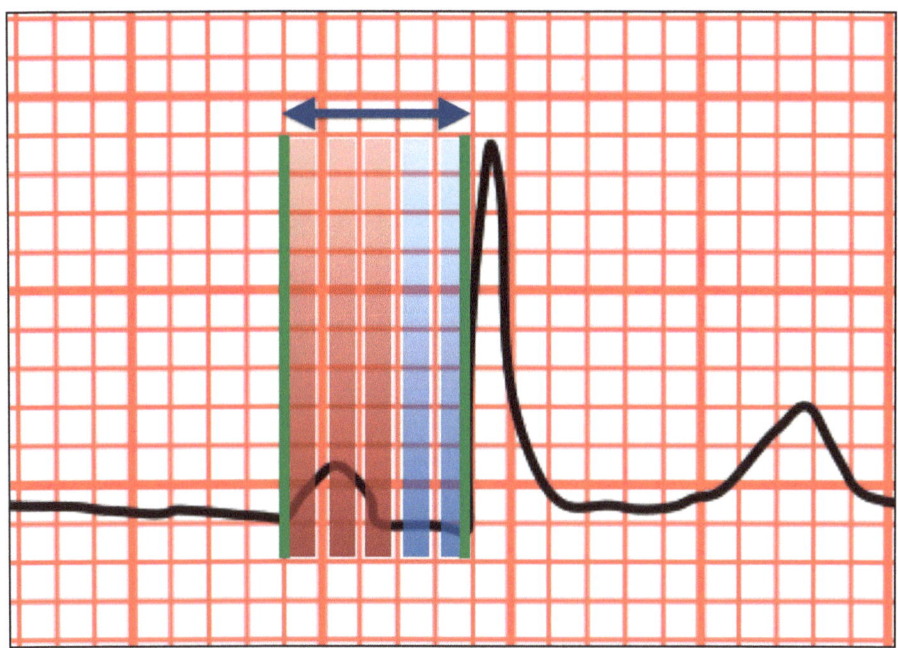

Step 3: 'P' Wave and Q'R'S Complex Relationship

In this rhythm, there's a **single P wave** before each **QRS complex**, and the *PR interval* is *normal*, less than 5 small squares.

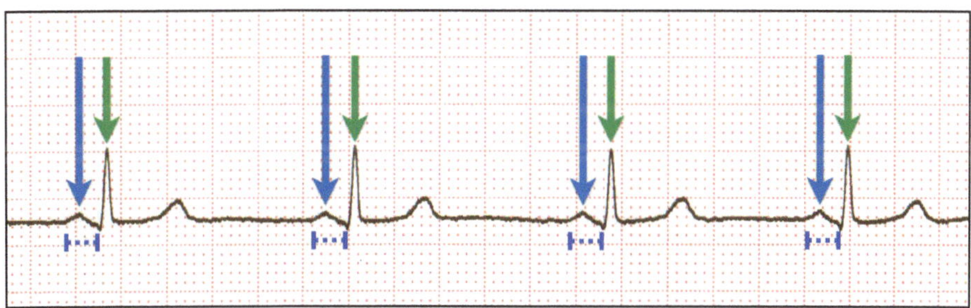

"In this rhythm analogy, imagine the **P wave** as the wife eagerly awaiting her husband, the **QRS complex**, to return home on time every day. In **sinus bradycardia**, their relationship is harmonious; he arrives promptly (**normal PR interval**), keeping their routine intact despite a slower pace."

"Tip: Follow '**R**' - '**Q**' - '**PR**' *pneumonic* when assessing a rhythm with brady (slow) rate. Example: **Rhythm: Regular, QRS: Narrow, PR interval: Normal = Sinus Bradycardia.**"

First Degree Heart Block

Step 1: Check Rhythm '*R*'egularity

The QRS complexes occur at evenly spaced intervals, confirming a steady and ***regular*** rhythm.

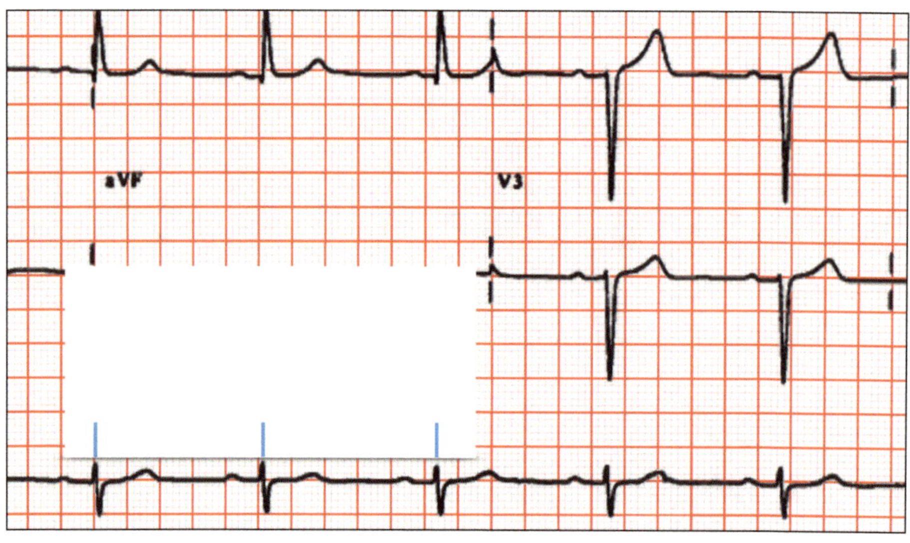

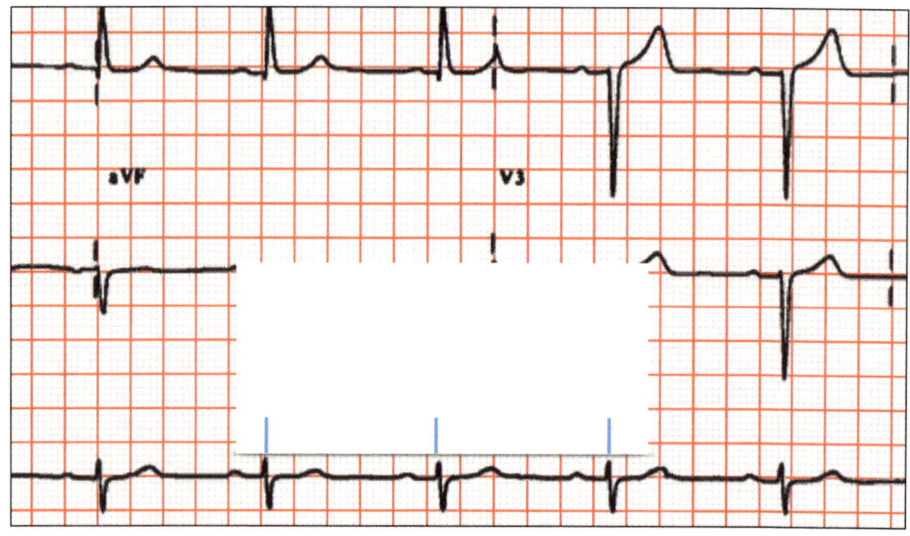

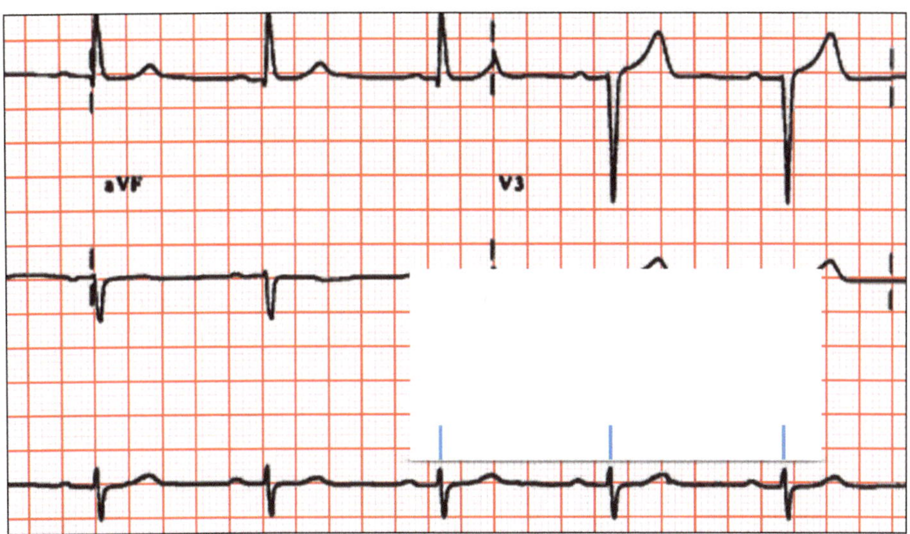

Step 2: 'Q'RS Width

The QRS complexes in this rhythm appear ***narrow***.

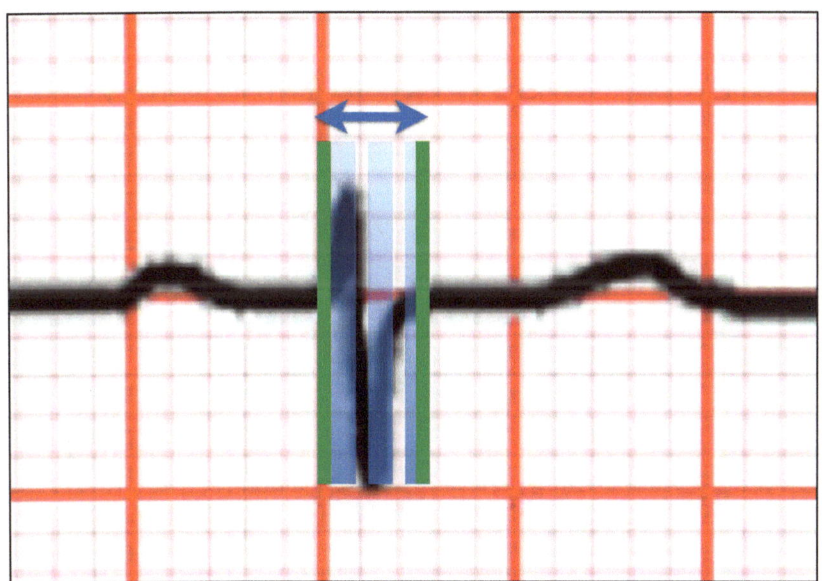

Step 3: '***P***' Wave and Q'***R***'S Complex Relationship

Similar to the previous rhythm, each **QRS complex** is preceded by a **single P wave**. However, in this case, the *PR interval* exceeds 5 small squares, indicating a *prolonged* duration.

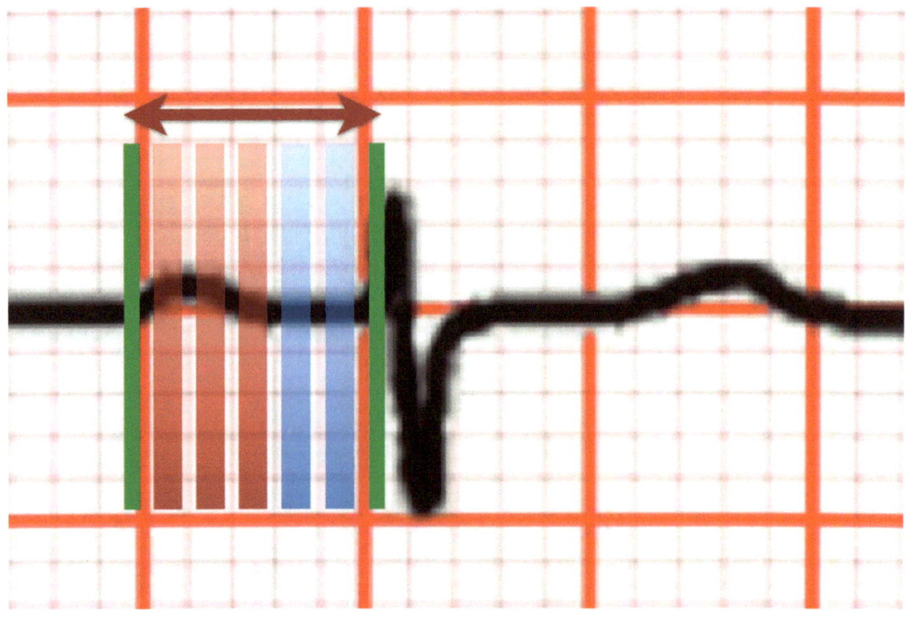

*"In **first-degree heart block**, after several years of marriage, the wife (**P wave**) patiently waits at home while the husband (**QRS complex**) returns home daily, but with a slight delay (**prolonged PR interval**)."*

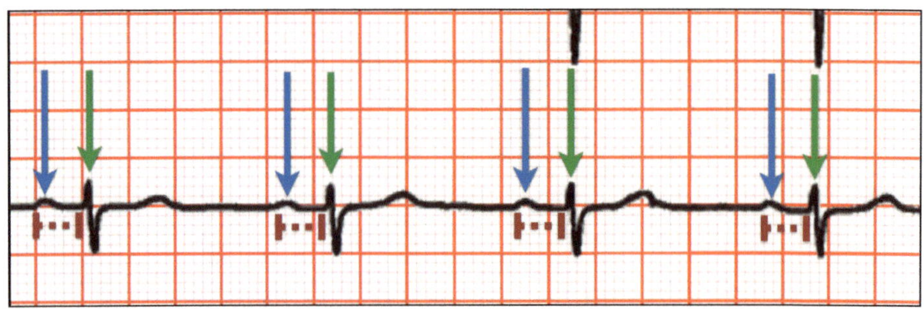

Rhythm:** Regular,* ***Q*RS: Narrow and* **PR** *interval: Prolonged = First degree heart block.*

Second Degree Type 1 Heart Block

Step 1: Check Rhythm **'R'**egularity

Here, we don't need a paper to see that the rhythm is **_irregular_**; it's evident just by looking.

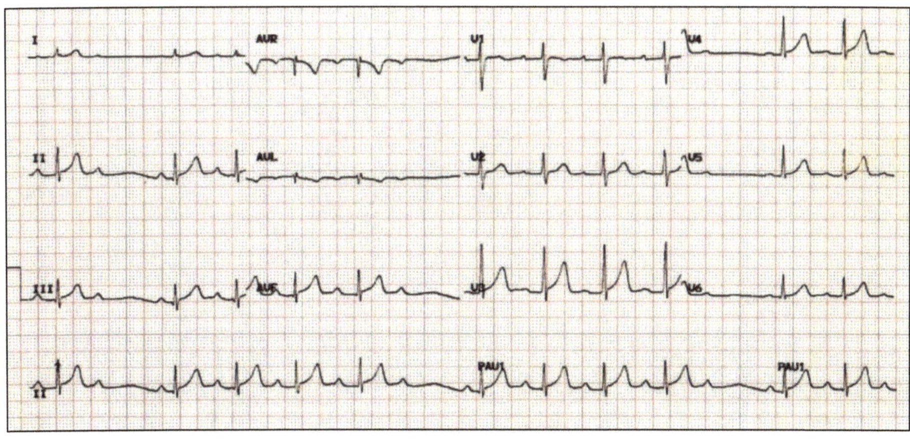

Step 2: **'Q'RS** Width

The QRS complex in this rhythm appears **_narrow_**.

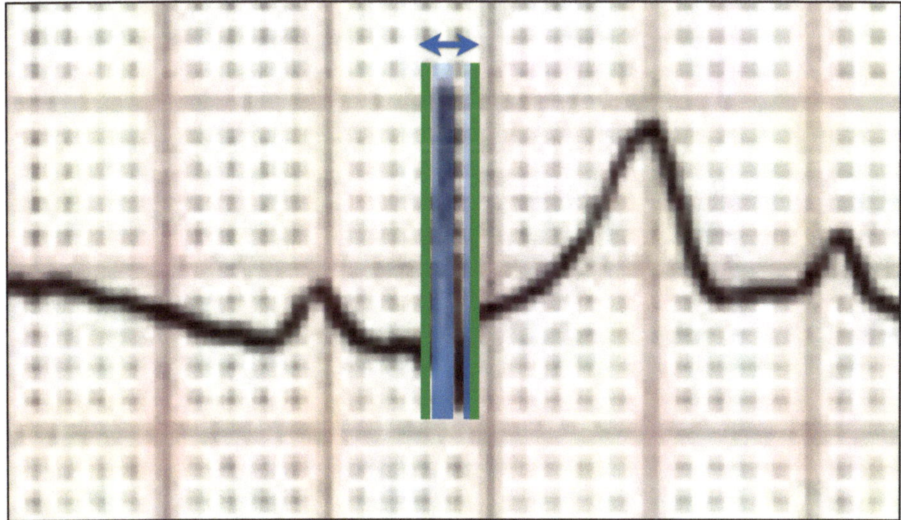

Step 3: '*P*' Wave and Q'*R*'S Complex Relationship

Something unique is occurring in this rhythm: with each successive beat, the *PR interval varies* and *progressively prolongs* until a QRS complex is **skipped**, restarting the cycle from a P wave. Consequently, there are more P waves than QRS complexes.

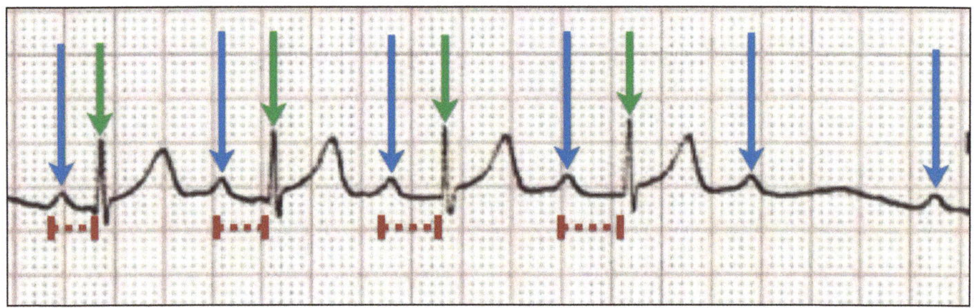

"In **second degree type 1 heart block (Mobitz type 1 /Wenckebach)**, *as the years of marriage pass, the wife (P wave) patiently waits at home while the husband (QRS complex) becomes increasingly erratic in his lateness, progressively delaying his return until one day he doesn't come home at all (PR prolongs and varies). This inconsistency causes tension and arguments, but they reconcile and the cycle restarts.*"

Rhythm: Irregular, **Q**RS: Narrow and **PR** interval: Prolonged = Second degree type 1 heart block.

Second Degree Type 2 Heart Block

Step 1: Check Rhythm '*R*'egularity

Just like with second-degree type 1 heart block, you can see right away that this rhythm is ***irregular***.

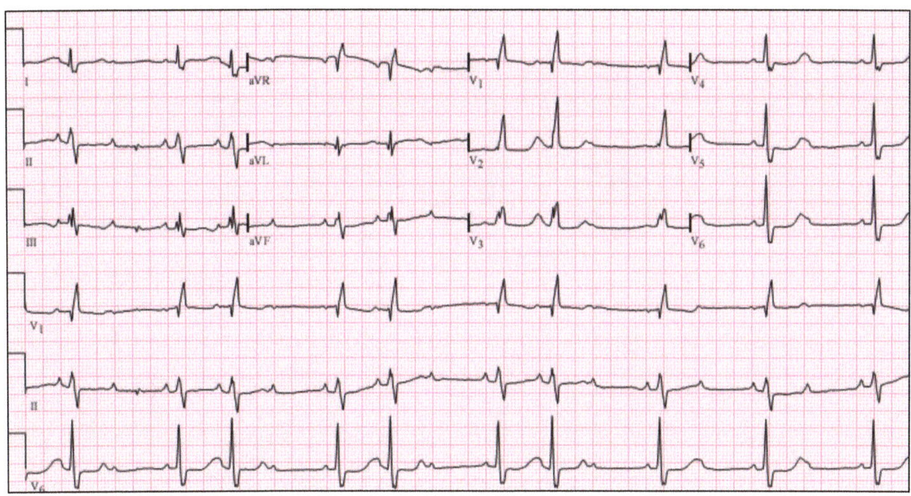

Step 2: 'Q'RS Width

Compared to the previous rhythm, the QRS complex in this rhythm is **wide**.

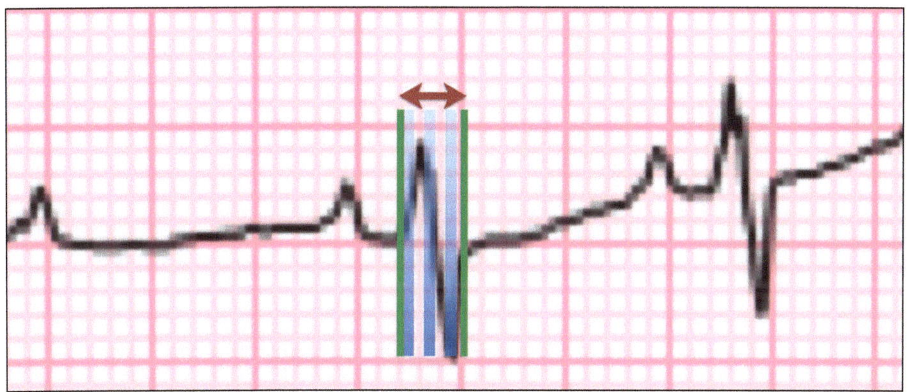

Step 3: 'P' Wave and Q'R'S Complex Relationship

Here, all the *PR intervals* are *fixed*, but intermittently, a **QRS complex** is **skipped**, restarting the cycle from the P wave. Consequently, in this rhythm as well, there are **more P waves** observed than QRS complexes.

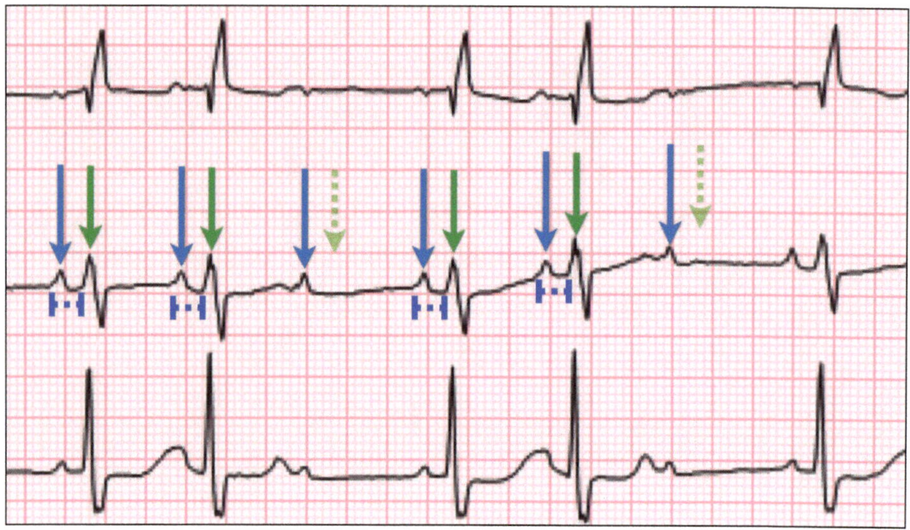

"*After a few more years of marriage, the wife (**P wave**) patiently waits at home while her husband (**QRS complex**) starts coming home regularly at a fixed time (**PR interval fixed**) for several days. However, unexpectedly, there are days when he doesn't return (**skipped QRS**). Each time this happens, his wife becomes deeply upset, leading to arguments, and the cycle repeats. This relationship resembles a **second-degree type 2 heart block**, also known as **Mobitz type 2 heart block.**"*

*Rhythm: Irregular, **QRS**: Wide and **PR** interval: Fixed = Second degree type 2 heart block.*

Third Degree Heart Block

Step 1: Check Rhythm '**R**'egularity

In this rhythm, the QRS complexes are equidistant, ensuring a **regular** rhythm similar to first-degree heart block.

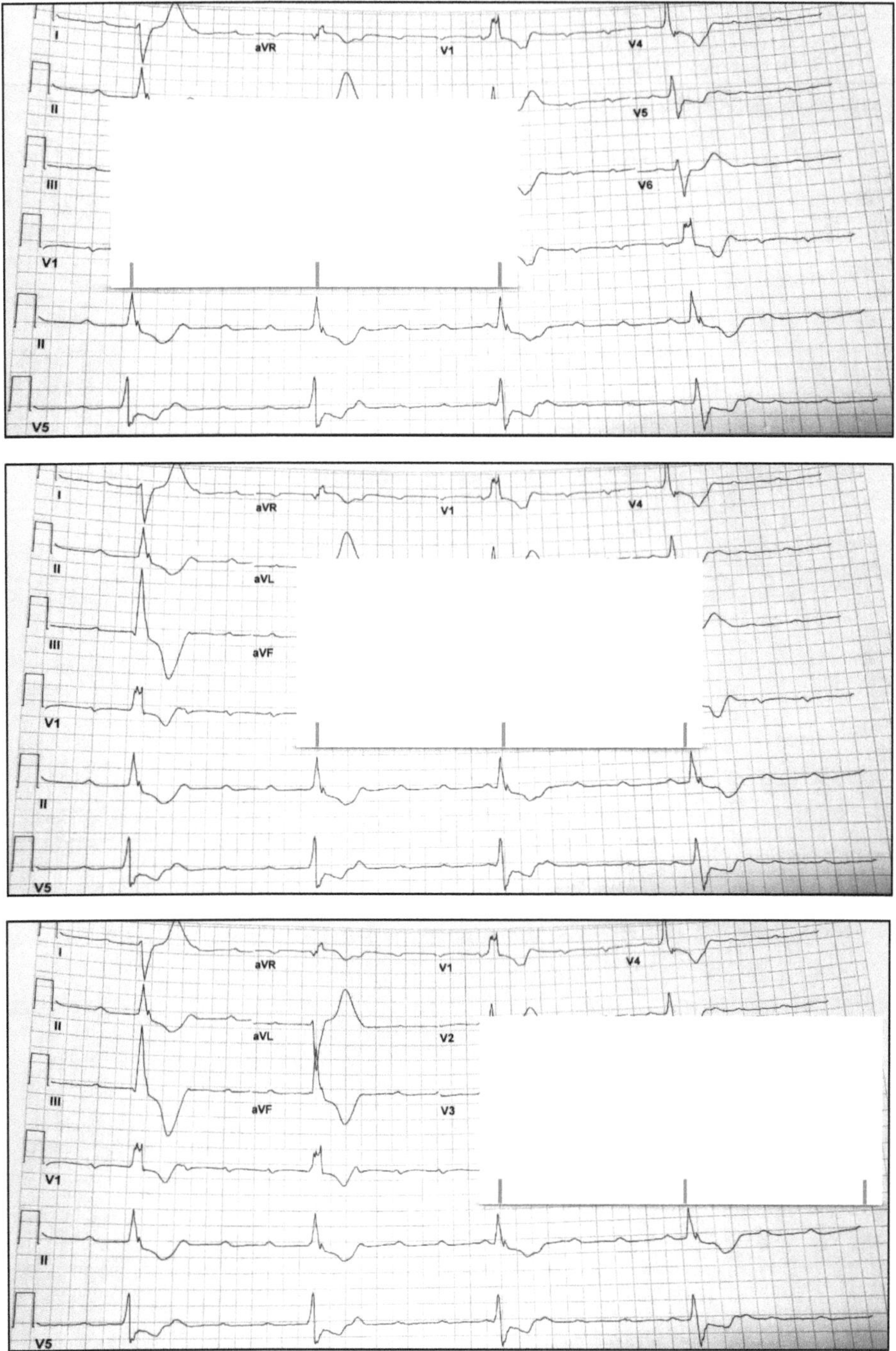

Step 2: 'Q'RS Width

Even without grid lines on ECG paper, it is evident that the QRS complexes in this rhythm are notably *wide*.

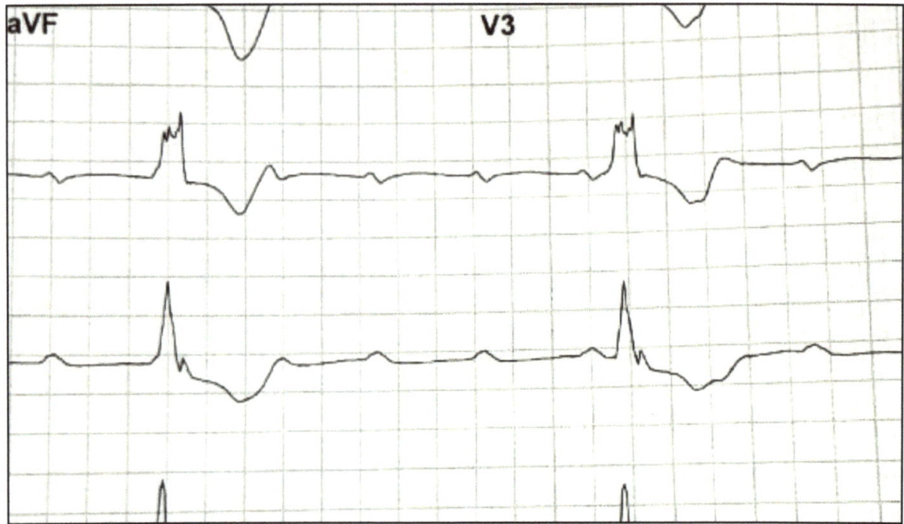

Step 3: 'P' Wave and Q'R'S Complex Relationship

Here, we observe a ***dissociation*** between P waves and QRS complexes. There is no consistent relationship between their timing. They proceed through the ECG at independent rates, with more P waves than QRS complexes present in this rhythm.

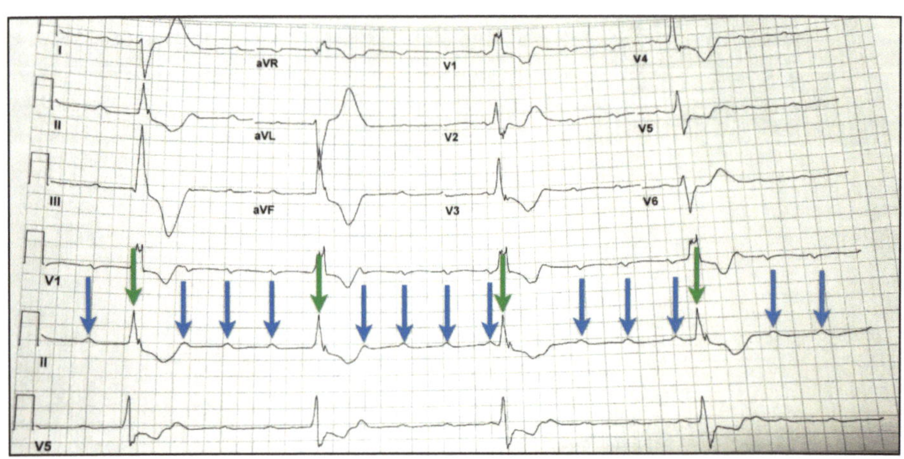

*"Finally, with no improvement in their relationship, the wife (**P wave**) stops waiting for the husband (**QRS complex**), who seems indifferent. Now, she leaves home and returns at her own pace, while the husband does the same. There is* **no coordination** *between them. This situation mirrors a* **third-degree heart block**, *also known as* **Complete Heart Block**.*"*

Rhythm: regular, **Q**RS: *Wide and* **P**-QRS: *Dissociation = Complete heart block.*

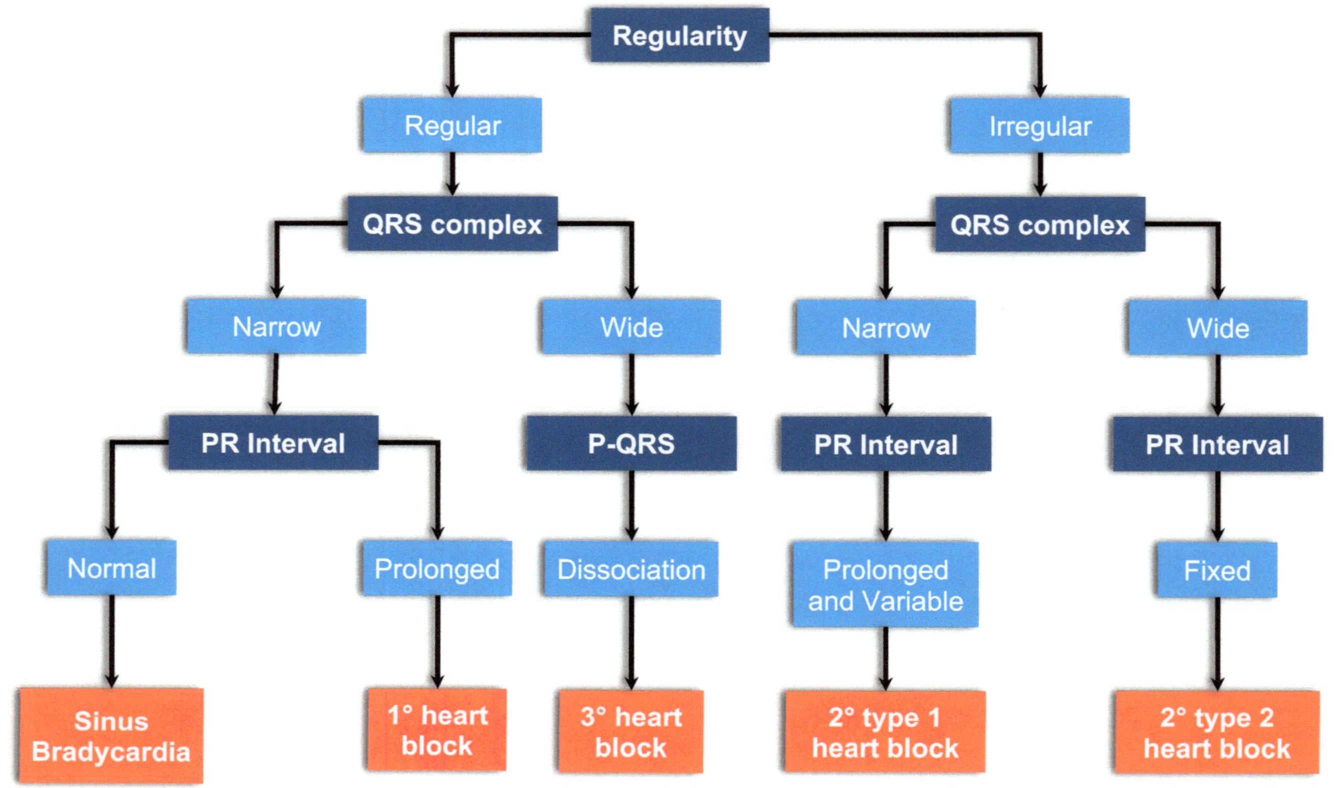

Regularity
Regular
Irregular
QRS complex
QRS complex
Narrow
Wide
Narrow
Wide
PR Interval
P-QRS
PR Interval
PR Interval
Normal
Prolonged
Dissociation
Prolonged and Variable
Fixed
Sinus Bradycardia
1° heart block
3° heart block
2° type 1 heart block
2° type 2 heart block

AXIS

Determining the cardiac axis from an ECG involves evaluating the direction of the QRS complex in lead I and lead aVF. The normal cardiac axis typically ranges between -30° and +90° in the vertical plane. Here's how you can identify different types of axis deviation:

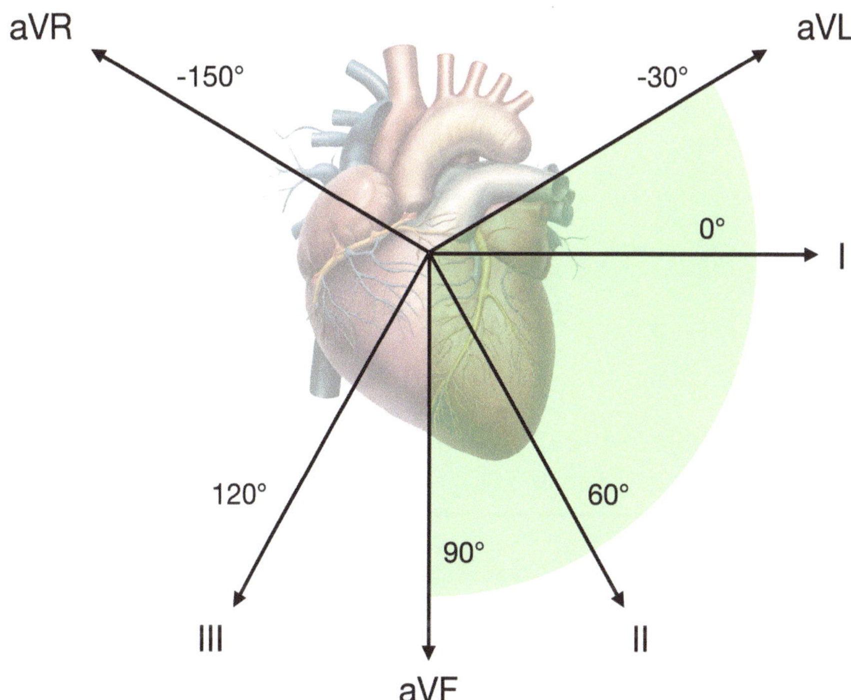

Normal Axis: Look at lead I and lead aVF. Imagine pointing your left thumb according to lead I's QRS direction and your right thumb according to lead aVF's QRS direction. If both thumbs point upwards (indicating predominantly positive QRS complexes in both leads), the axis is considered normal.

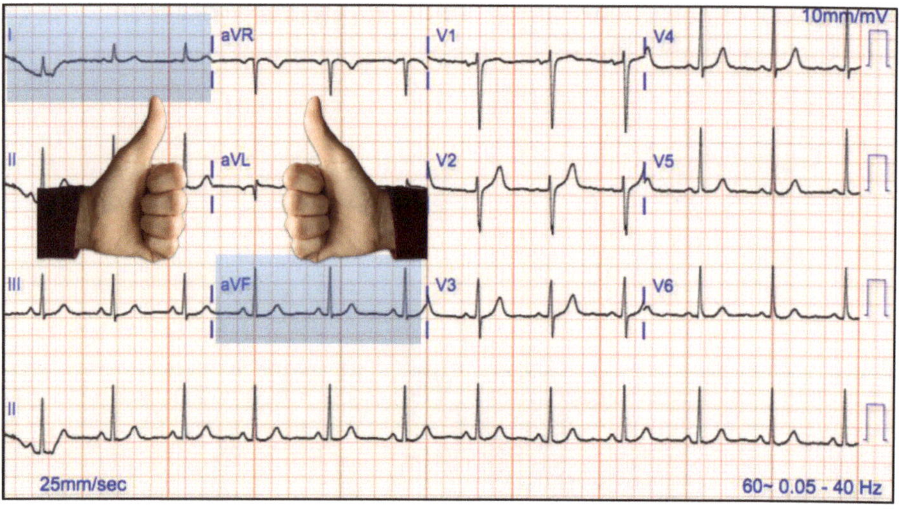

Left Axis Deviation (LAD): In lead I, the QRS complex is upright (left thumb up), while in lead aVF, it points downward (right thumb down).

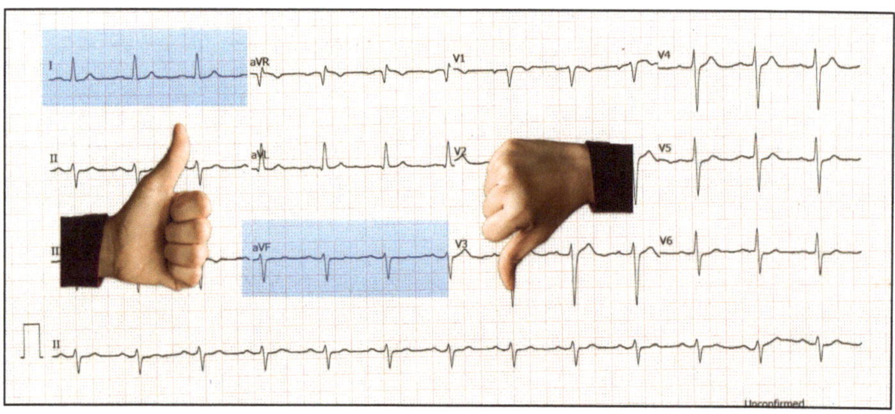

When you place your hands one above the other (left hand above right), both thumbs point away from each other (*Left axis deviation = Leaves*), indicating a leftward shift of the cardiac axis.

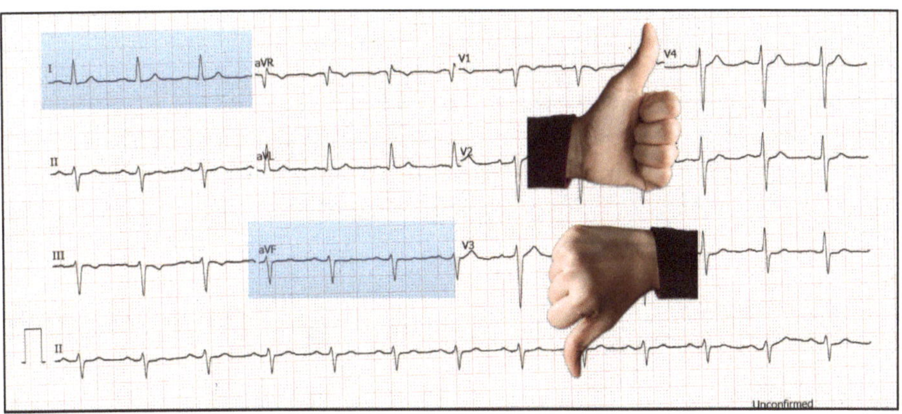

Right Axis Deviation (RAD): In lead I, the QRS complex is downward (left thumb down), and in lead aVF, it is upward (right thumb up).

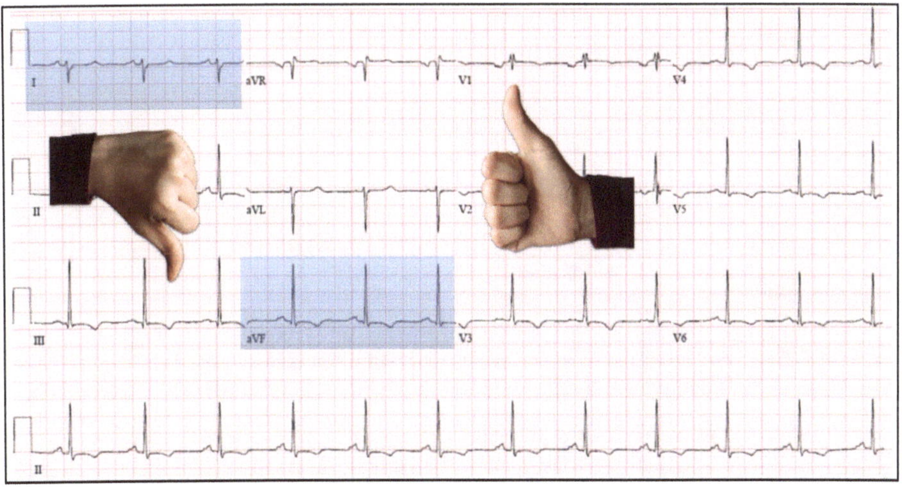

Placing your left hand (thumb down) over your right hand (thumb up), you'll notice both thumbs facing each other *(**Right axis deviation** = **Returns**)*, indicating a rightward shift of the cardiac axis.

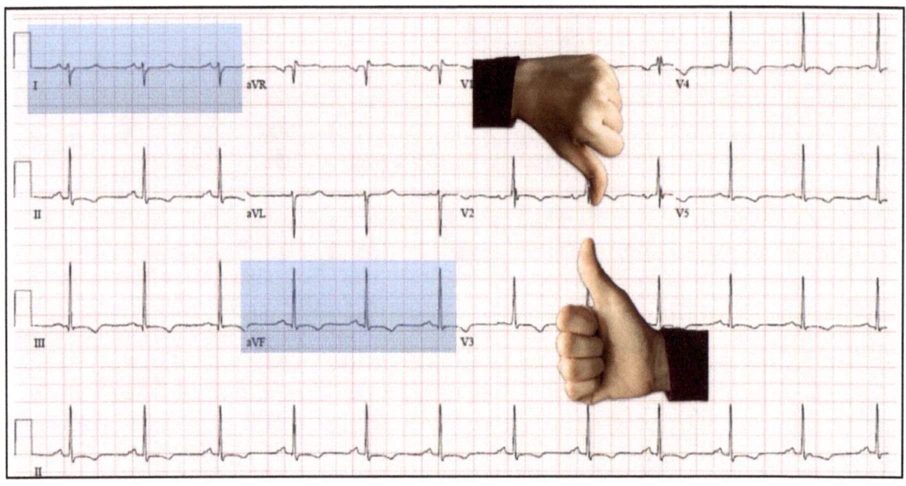

Extreme Axis Deviation (EAD): Both lead I and lead aVF show downward-pointing QRS complexes (both thumbs down), suggesting an extreme deviation of the cardiac axis.

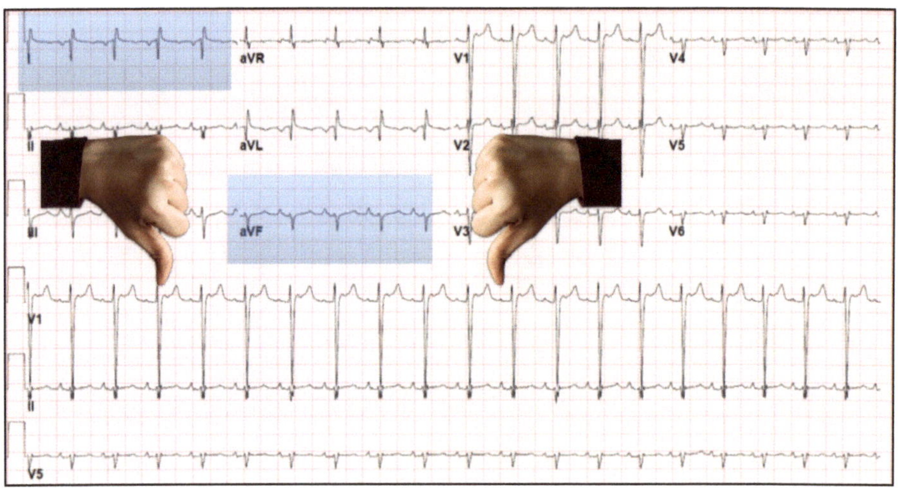

WAVES, SEGMENTS AND INTERVALS

Having covered the QRS complex and PR interval in our previous discussion on rhythm, let's now explore other waves, segments, and intervals in electrocardiography.

Any deviation from the baseline is identified as a **wave**, such as the P wave, QRS complex, and T wave.

A **segment** refers to the straight line between two waves on the ECG, for instance, the ST segment found between the QRS complex and T wave.

An **interval** comprises a segment along with one or more waves. For example, the PR interval includes the P wave and the PR segment.

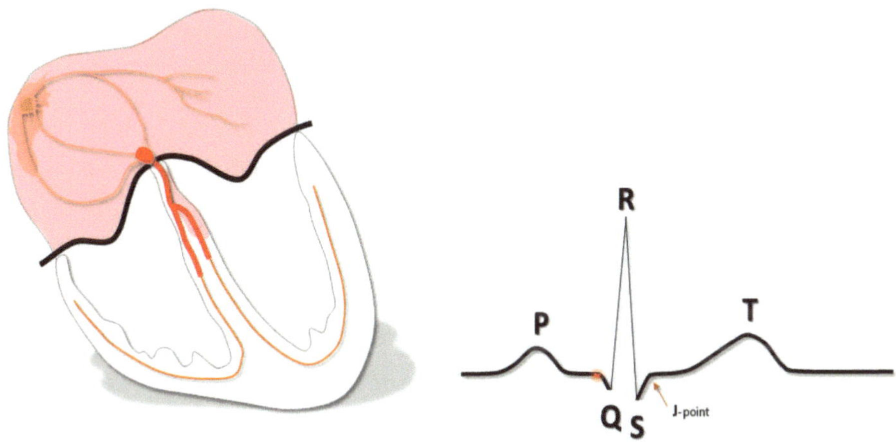

Understanding these definitions is crucial for accurately interpreting the various components of an ECG, which is essential for diagnosing and understanding cardiac conditions.

P Wave

The best lead to observe P waves is lead II. A normal P wave typically measures less than 3 small squares in height and width.

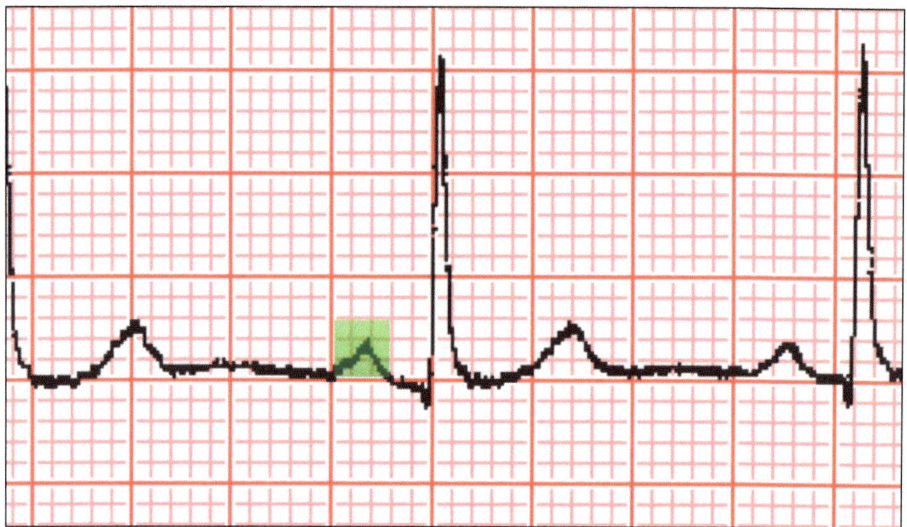

A tall P wave exceeding 3 small squares in height is termed 'P pulmonale' suggestive of **right atrial enlargement**, while a P wave wider than 3 small squares is known as 'P mitrale' suggestive of **left atrial enlargement**.

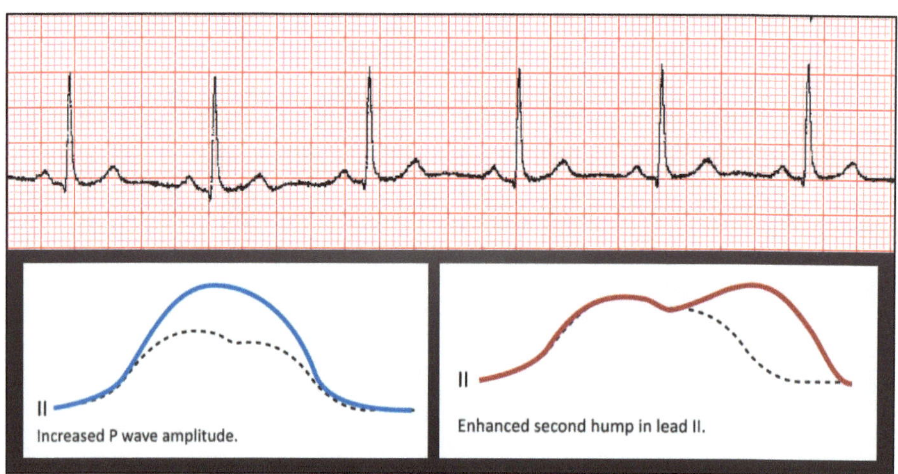

As compared to the normal P waves, the P waves in the bottom strip appear tall and **peaked,** suggestive of **P pulmonale**. *(Peaked = Pulmonale).*

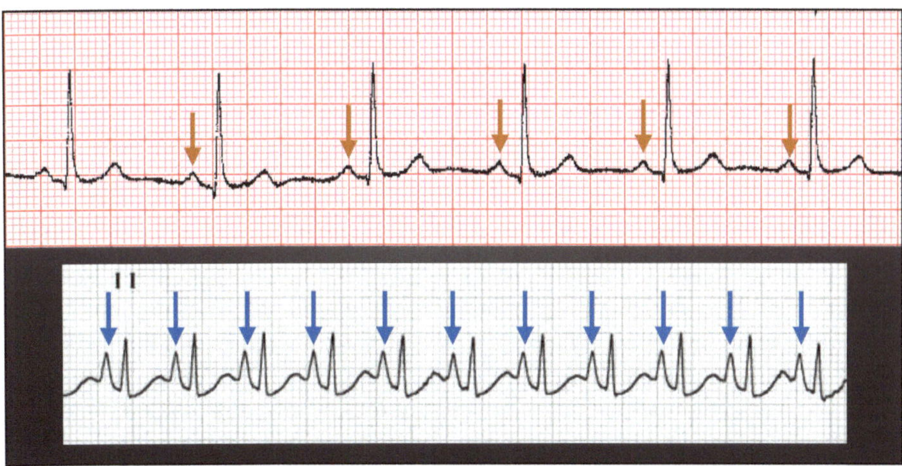

Compared with the normal P waves, the P waves in the bottom strip appear wide and **'M' shaped**, indicative of **P mitrale**. *('M' shaped = Mitrale).*

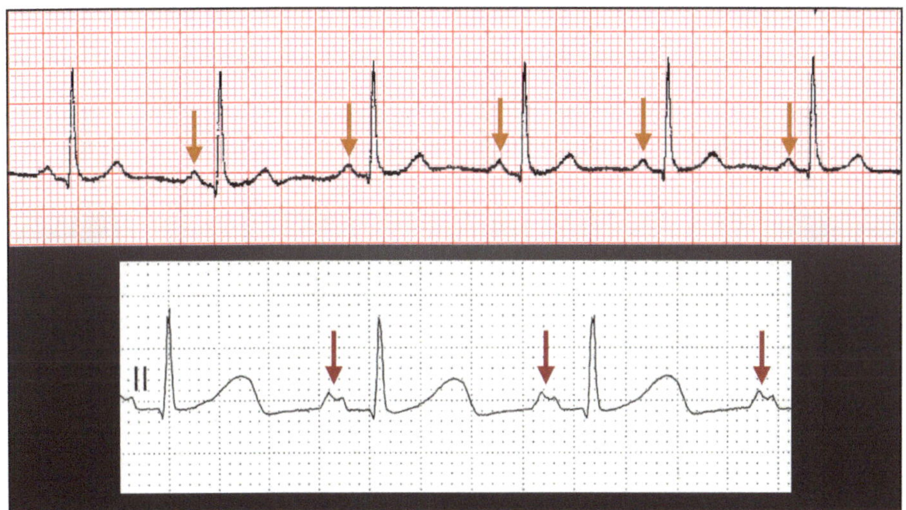

ST Segment

The ST segment on an ECG is the line that connects the end of the QRS complex to the start of the T wave.

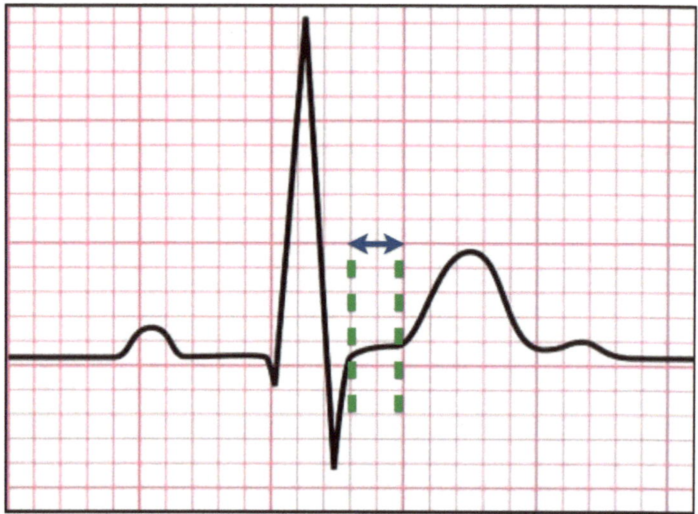

We can **use the PR segment** (the line from the end of the P wave to the beginning of the QRS complex) **as a baseline** to assess any elevation or depression of the ST segment.

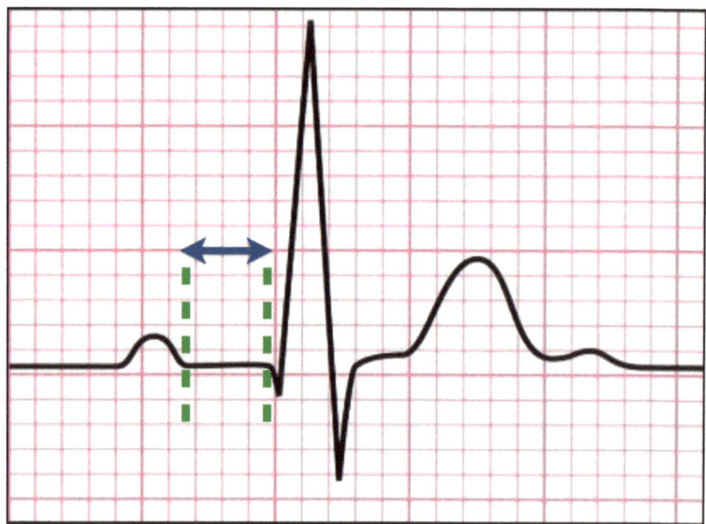

The ST segment elevation or depression is measured at the J Point, which is the junction point between the QRS complex and the ST segment. This measurement is compared to the **baseline** provided by the PR segment.

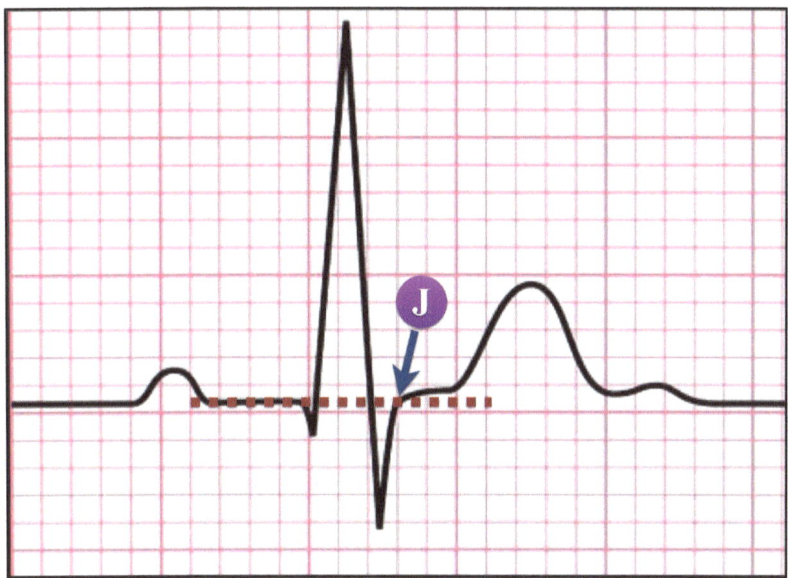

The ECG uses multiple leads to measure electrical activity from different angles of the heart. Leads that are positioned next to one another and record activity from the same region of the heart are called **contiguous (neighbouring) leads**. For example:

- **Leads V1-V4** are contiguous and primarily reflect activity in the **anterior wall** of the heart.

- **Leads II, III, and aVF** are contiguous and focus on the **inferior wall**.

- **Leads I, aVL, V5, and V6** are contiguous, representing the **lateral wall**.

The presence of ST segment deviation is clinically significant only if it is there in **at least two contiguous leads,** strengthening the possibility of a specific cardiac abnormality. For instance, ST elevation in multiple contiguous leads of a specific region might suggest a heart attack in that area.

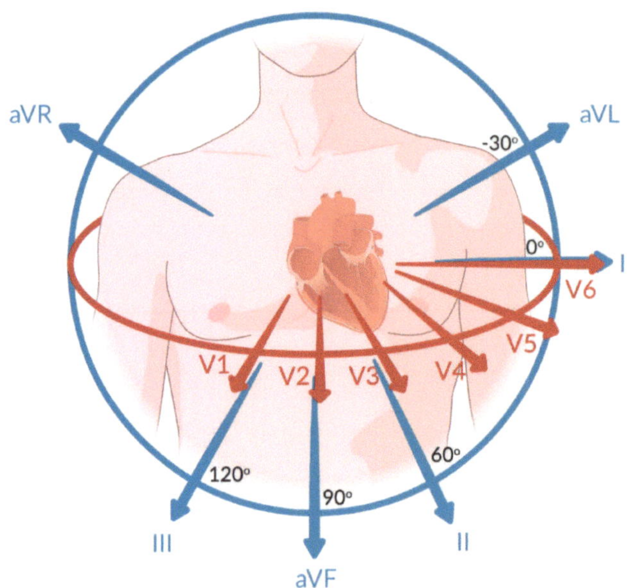

To practically interpret ST deviations on the ECG, we categorize the leads as follows:

- Leads V1 to V4: Anteroseptal

- Leads I, aVL, V5, V6: Lateral

- Leads II, III, and aVF: Inferior

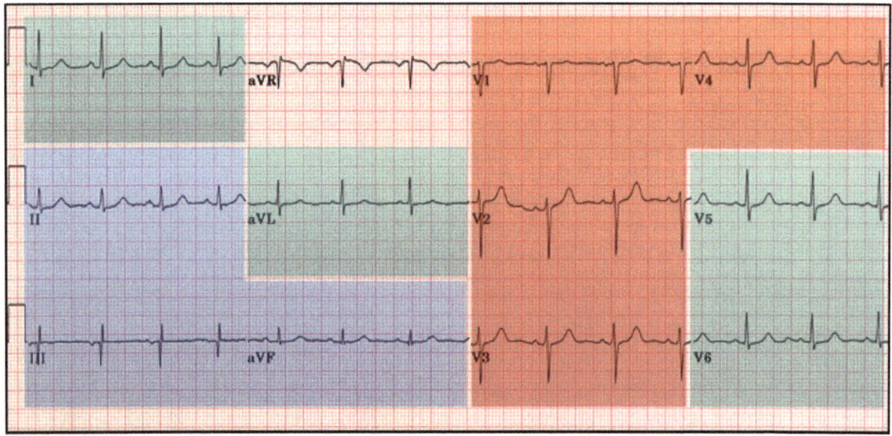

To measure ST elevation accurately, first identify the PR segment (**baseline**) on the ECG.

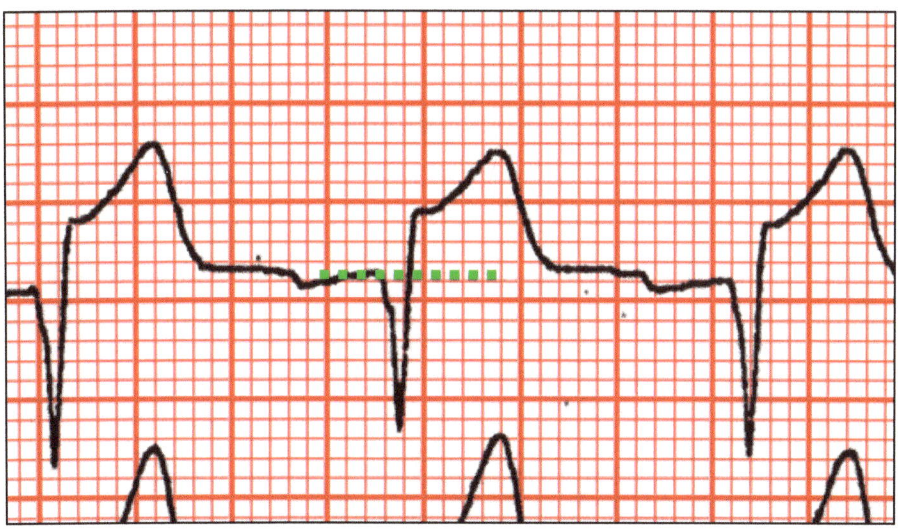

Once you locate the **baseline** (you can use a small piece of paper to mark it), count the number of small squares above it to the **J point**. If the **elevation exceeds 1 small square** in any lead (except leads V2 and V3, where it should exceed 2 small squares), **it is considered significant. If ST elevations are present in at least two contiguous leads, it could indicate a STEMI (ST-segment elevation myocardial infarction).**

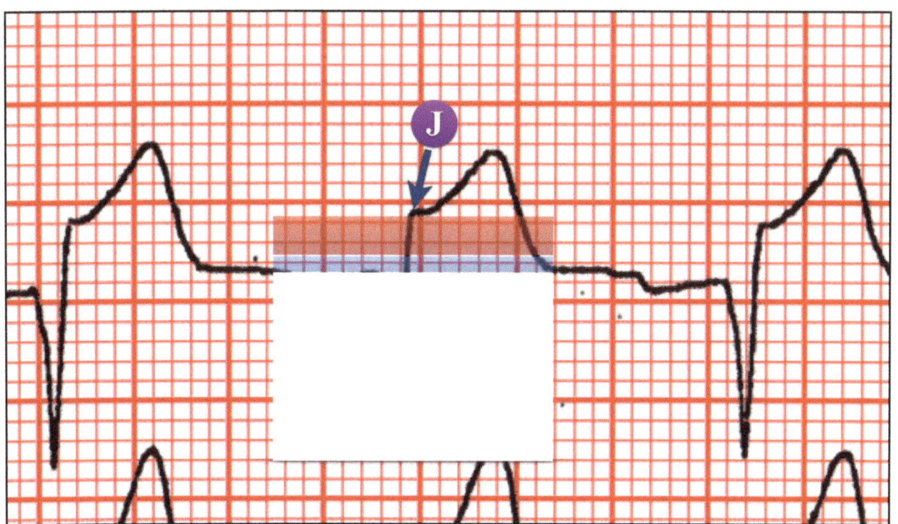

Similarly, to measure ST depression, begin by identifying the PR segment (baseline) on the ECG.

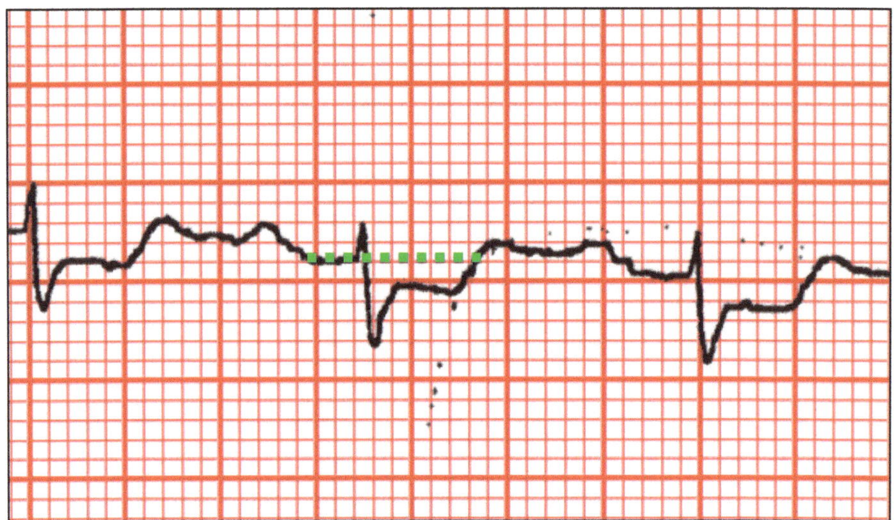

In case of ST depression, count the number of small squares below it to the J point on the ECG. If the **depression exceeds half a small square in any lead, it is considered significant**. This finding gains clinical importance **if ST depressions are present in at least two contiguous leads,** which **could indicate acute coronary syndrome (ACS).**

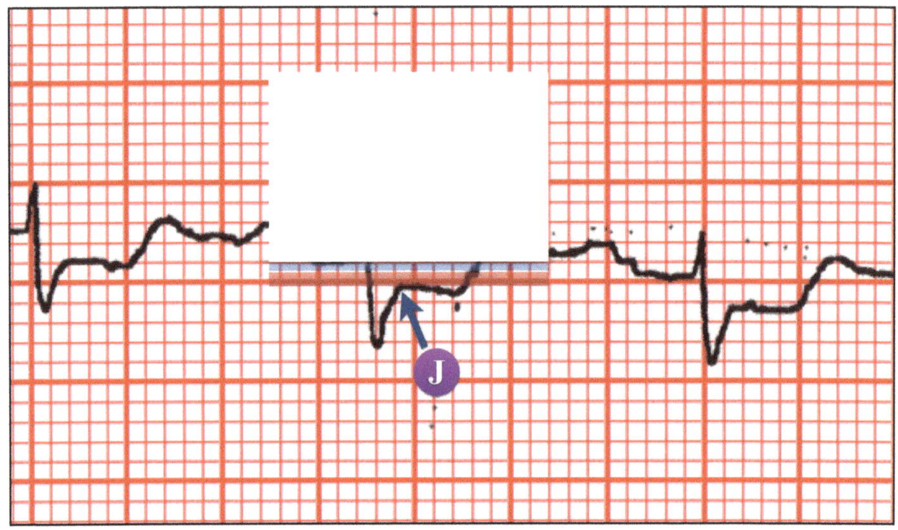

In the following ECG, significant **ST elevations** are observed in the contiguous anterior leads V1 to V3, as well as in the lateral leads I and aVL, indicative of an **Anterolateral STEMI**. In contrast, there are **reciprocal ST depressions** noted in the inferior leads II, III, and aVF. These changes are expected in Anterolateral STEMI due to the anatomical relationship where the inferior leads view the heart from an almost opposite angle to the anterolateral leads.

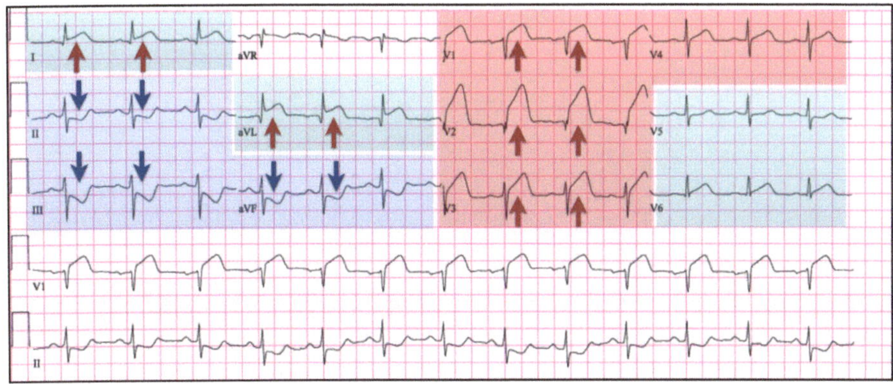

In the following ECG, significant **ST elevations** are observed in the contiguous inferior leads II, III, and aVF, indicative of an **Inferior wall STEMI**. Additionally, there is a **reciprocal ST depression** noted in the lateral lead aVL, consistent with the anatomical relationship where changes in inferior leads can produce reciprocal changes in lateral leads.

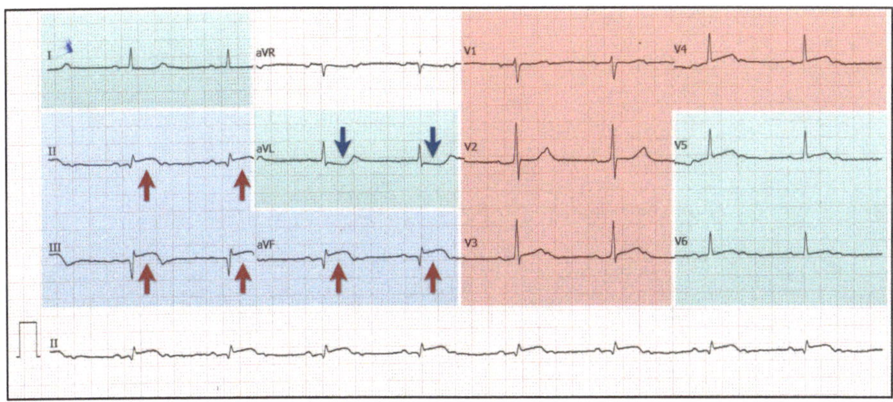

Till now, we have discussed three territories for ST deviation: inferior, anteroseptal, and lateral. However, there is another important territory to consider. In this ECG, significant **ST depressions** are observed particularly **in leads V1 to V3**. These findings represent reciprocal ST depressions, as we discussed earlier. The presence of ST depressions in these anterior precordial leads suggests involvement of the posterior territory, which is anatomically opposite to these leads.

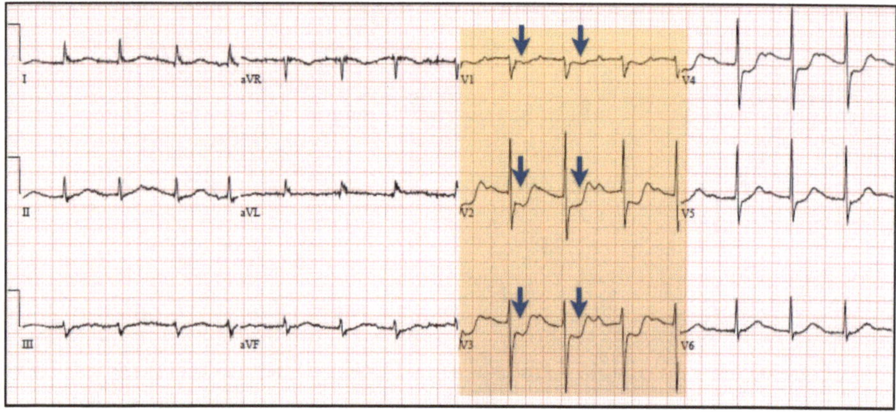

Tip: If you observe ST depressions in leads V1 to V3 on an ECG, try flipping the ECG and viewing it against a light source. When viewed from the blank side, you'll notice that the tracing appears faint, but the ST depressions will now appear as ST elevations. This change can suggest possible **ST elevation** *in the posterior leads, providing a hint towards posterior* **myocardial infarction.**"

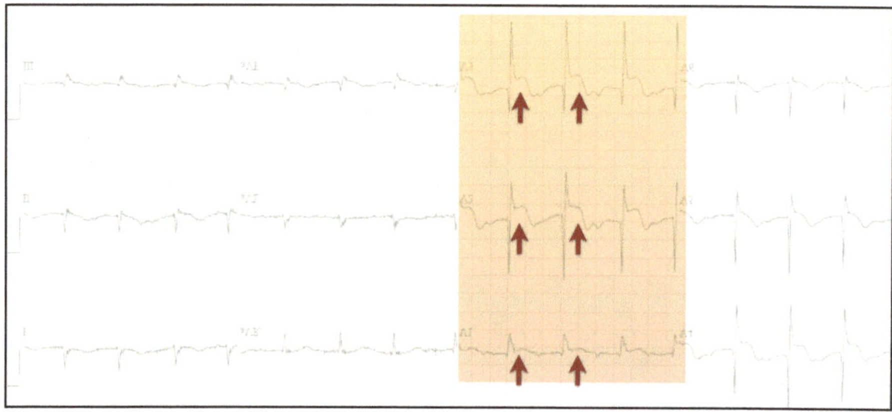

To confirm this, remove the electrodes V4, V5, and V6 and reattach them at **positions V7, V8, and V9** respectively (**posterior electrodes**), as shown in the diagram, and record the ECG again.

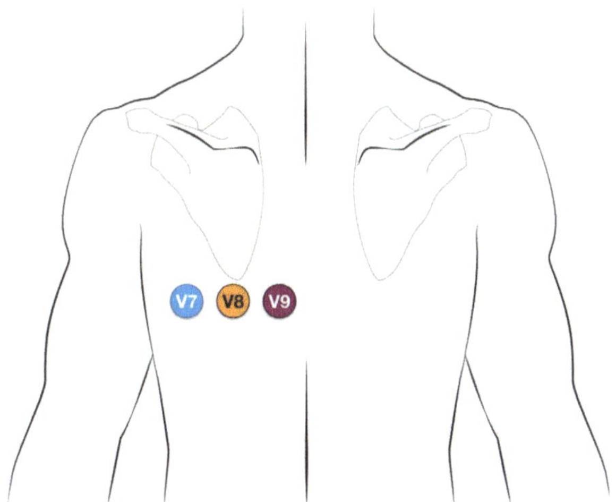

If there are **ST elevations of more than half a small square in at least two contiguous posterior leads** (V8 and V9 in this case), it is indicative of a **Posterior wall STEMI**.

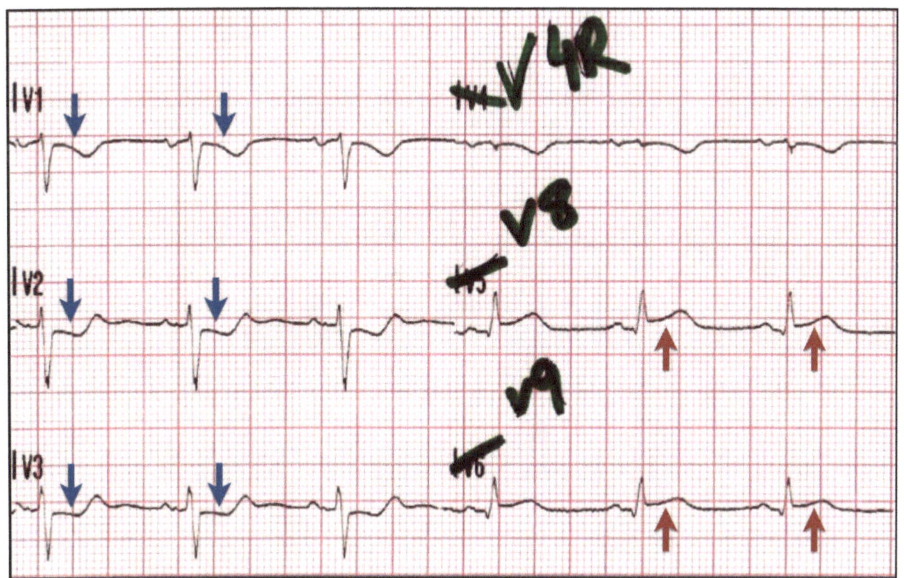

T Wave

The normal T wave typically measures less than 1 large square in height in limb leads and less than 2 large squares in height in chest leads.

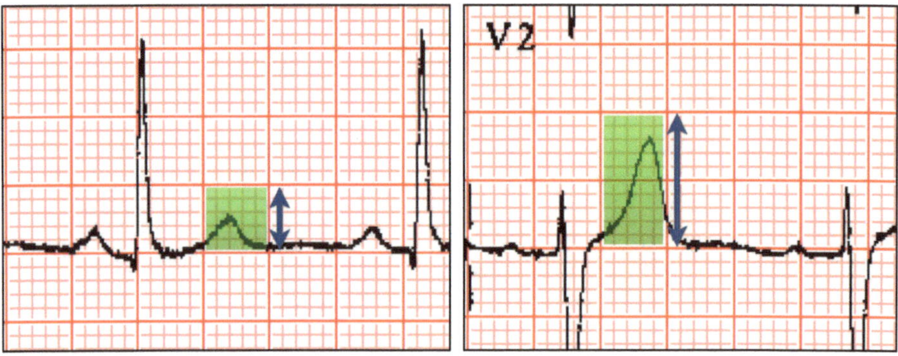

Tall and 'curved' T waves are referred to as **hyper-acute T waves** and are characteristic findings seen in the **early stages of STEMI** when present in two or more contiguous leads.

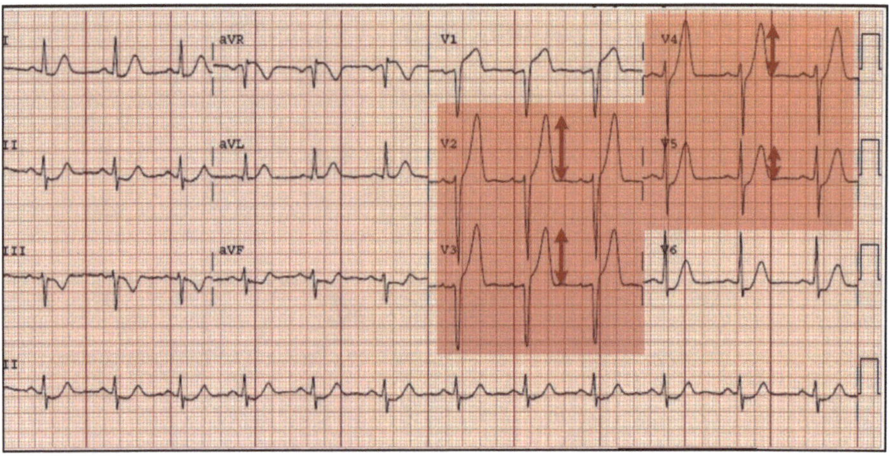

Another variant is **tall and 'peaked' T waves**, which are characteristic findings **observed in hyperkalemia**.

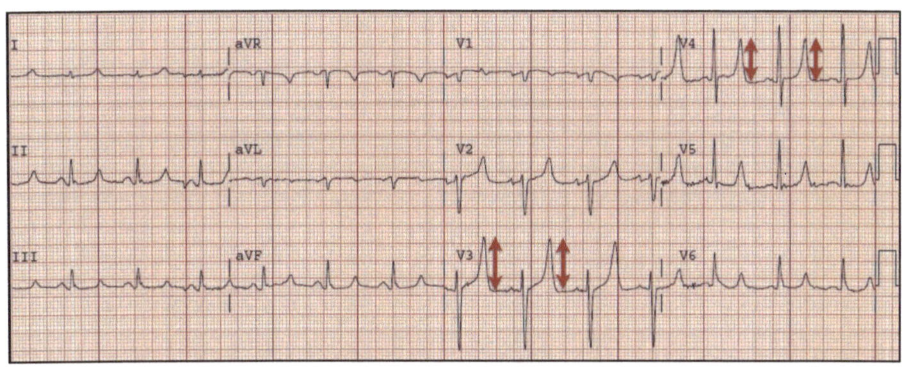

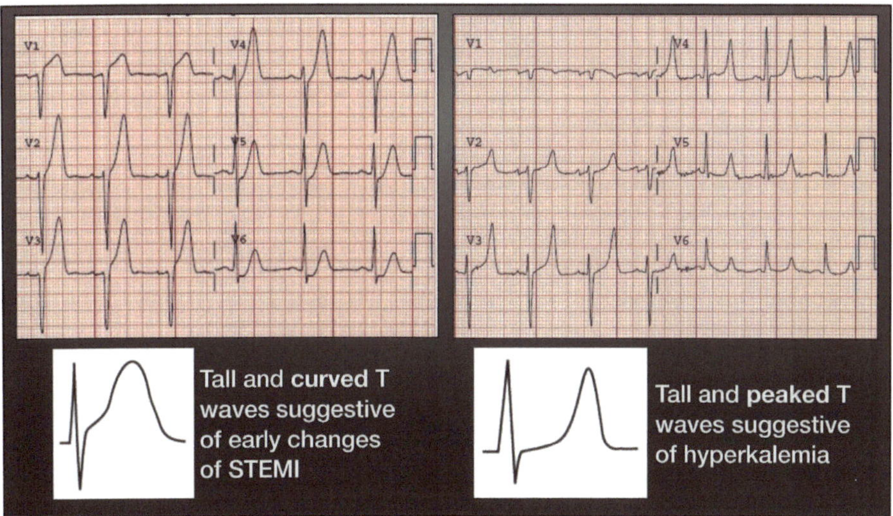

QT Interval

The QT interval spans from the onset of the QRS complex to the end of the T wave. Lead II is considered the optimal lead for measuring the QT interval. The QT interval varies and is inversely proportional to the heart rate. **Prolonged QT interval is associated with an increased risk of fatal arrhythmias.**

By definition, **a normal QT interval** is typically **less than half of the preceding RR interval** (the distance between two QRS complexes). **If the QT interval exceeds this duration, it is considered prolonged.**

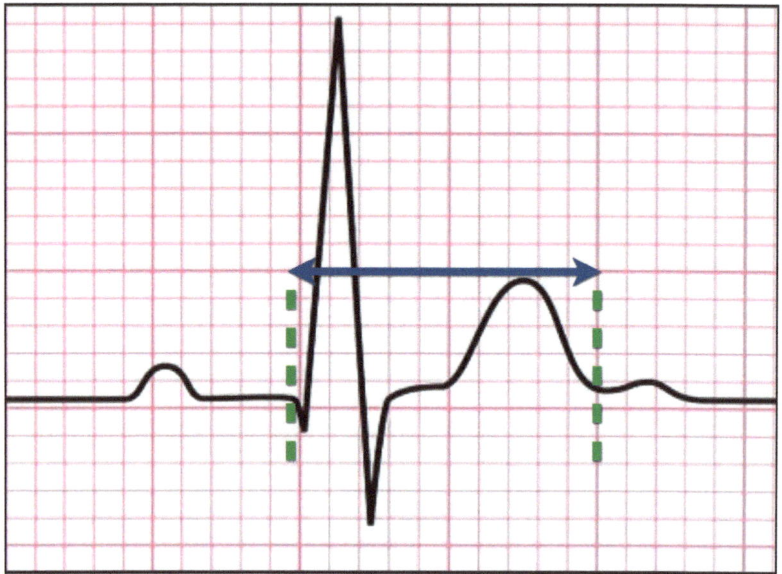

If the rhythm is regular, the current RR interval and the preceding RR interval will be identical. Therefore, if the QT interval is less than half of the current RR interval, it is considered normal; if it exceeds this duration, it is considered prolonged.

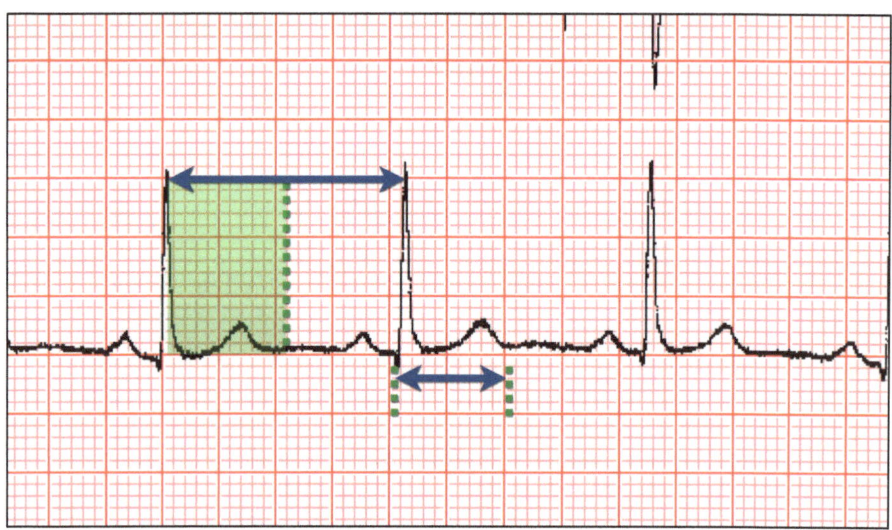

Tip: *To see this practically on ECG, fold the ECG paper to join the tips of two adjacent QRS complexes, creating a crease in between that represents*

half of the RR interval. If the end of the T wave extends beyond this crease, it indicates a prolonged QT interval

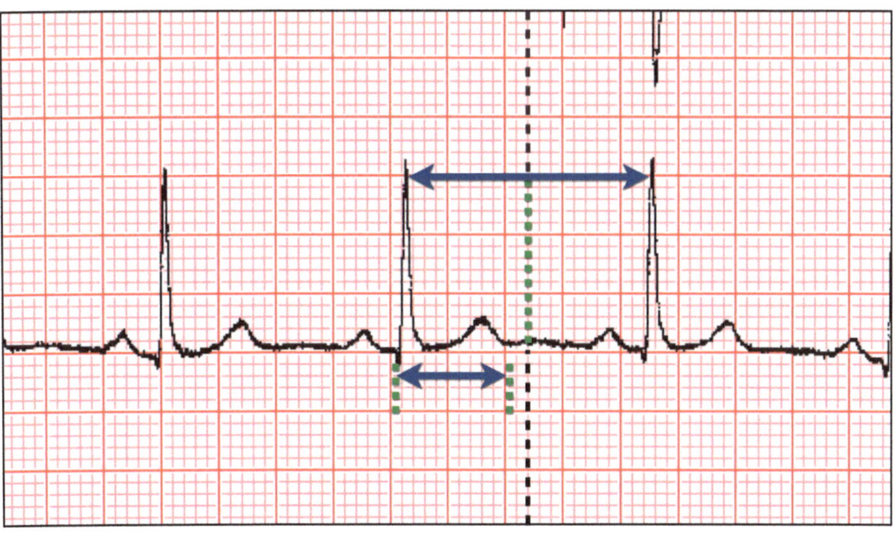

SUMMARY

1. Check Identification

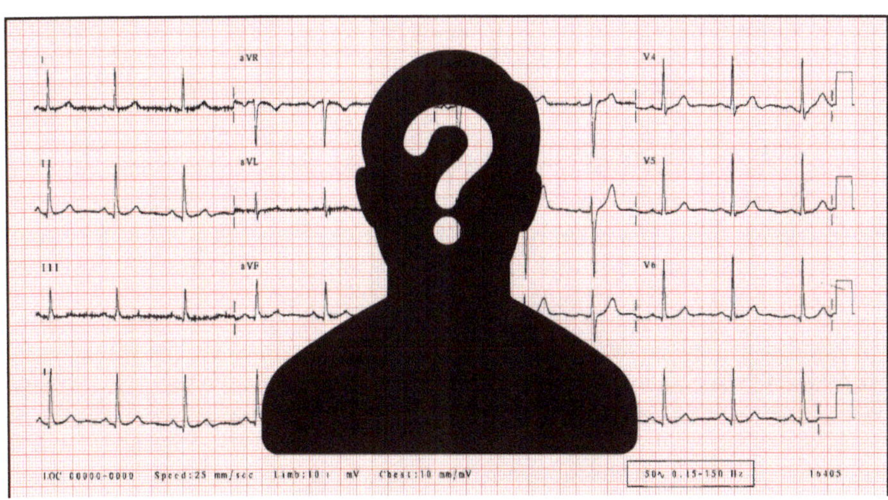

2. Check Validity

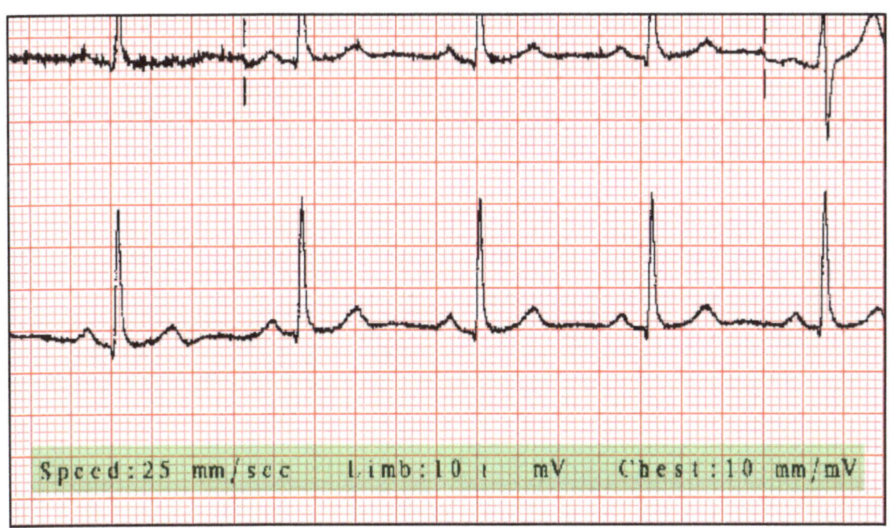

- *Standard Calibration: 25 mm/sec, 10 mm / mV*

- *Electrode Placement:* Check leads I, II and III for all inverted waves or near flat line.

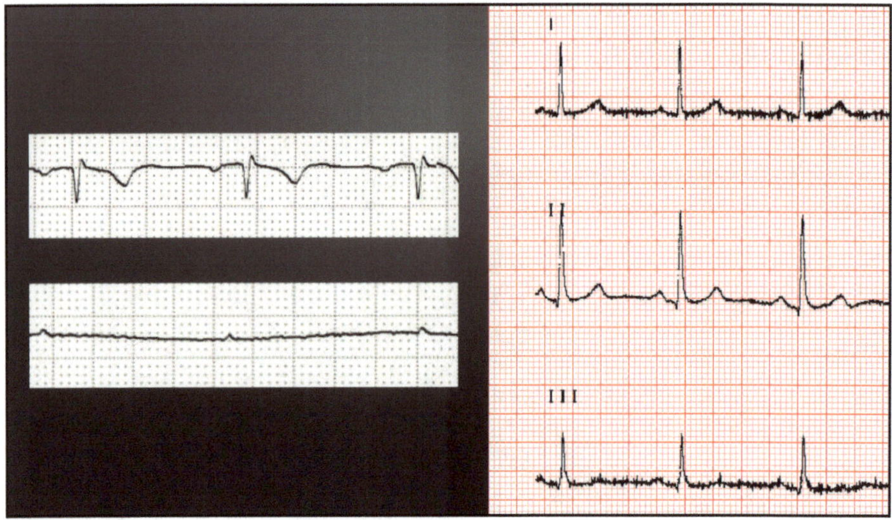

3. ***Check Rate:*** Count number of QRS complexes in rhythms strip and multiply by 6.

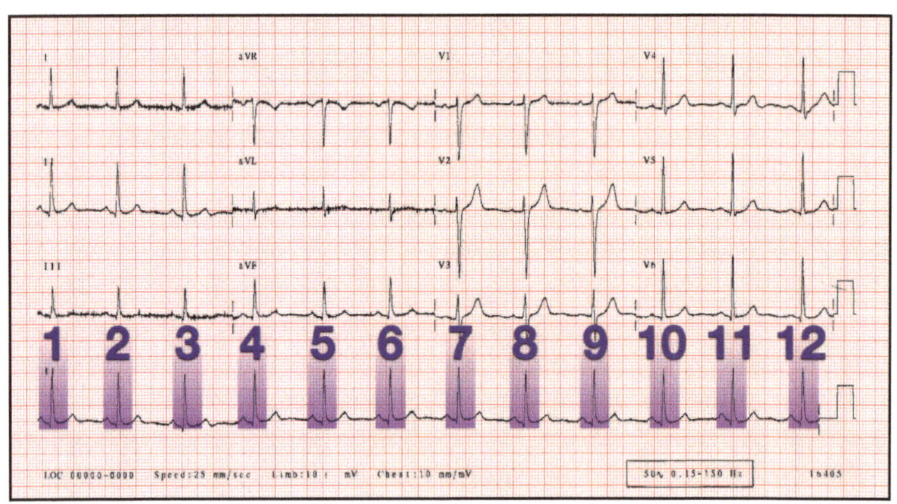

4. *Check Rhythm:* R-Q-P for fast rhythms, R-Q-PR for slow rhythms

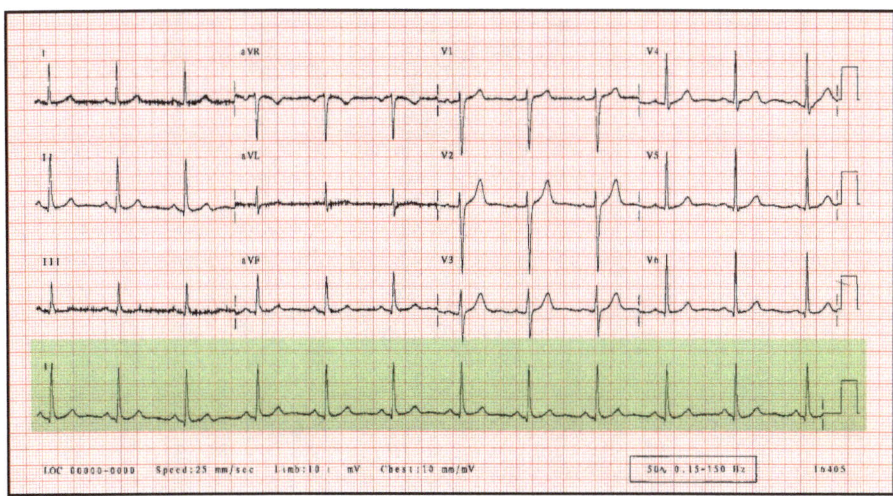

- *QRS Complex:* Less than 3 small squares wide is normal.

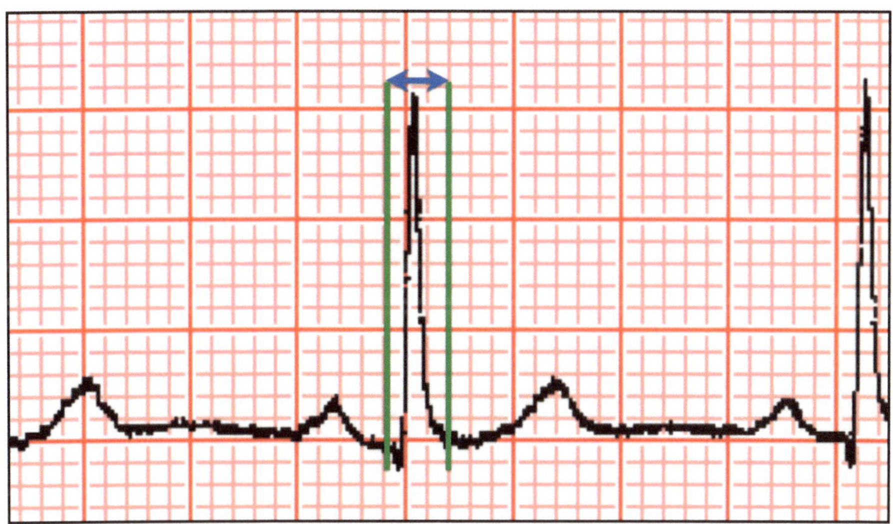

- *PR Interval:* 3 to 5 small squares duration is normal.

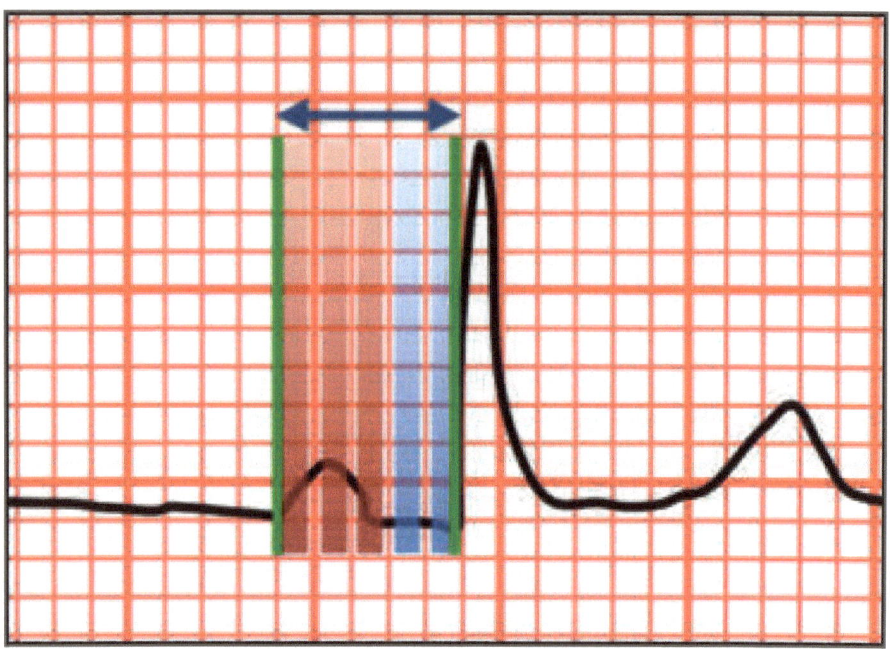

5. *Check Axis:* QRS pointing up in both lead I and aVF is normal.

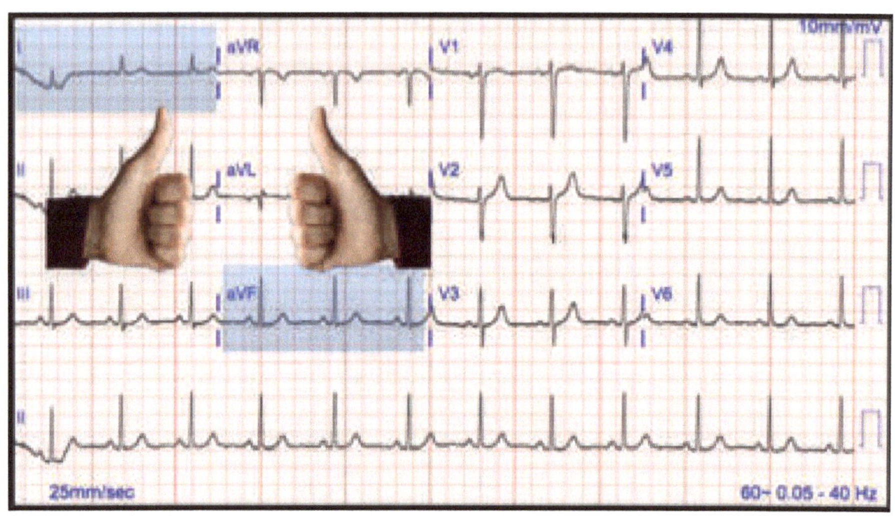

6. Check Waves, Segments and Intervals

- *P Wave:* Normally it is 3 X 3 small squares in height and width

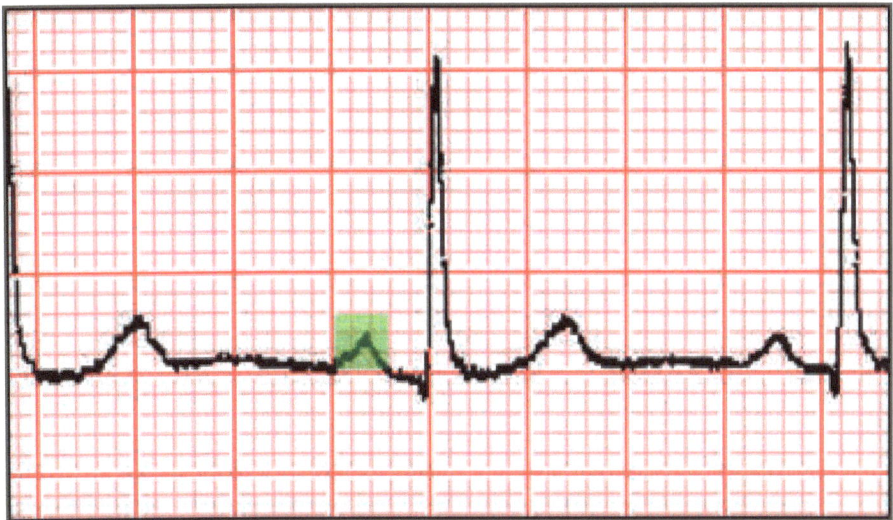

- *ST Segment:* ST elevation more than 1 small square and ST depression more than half small square in any lead is significant.

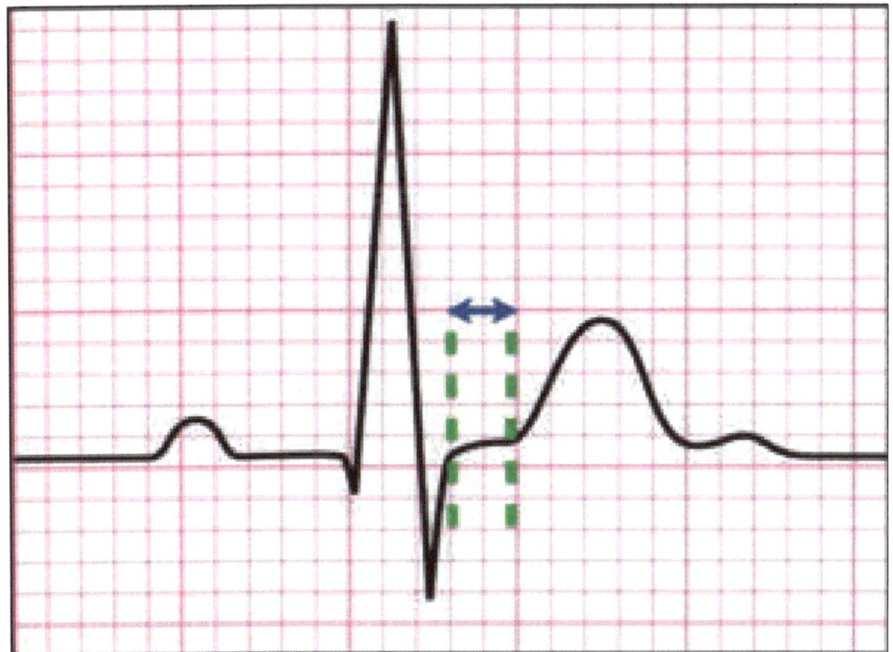

- *T Wave:* Height of less than 1 large square in limb leads and 2 large squares in chest leads is normal.

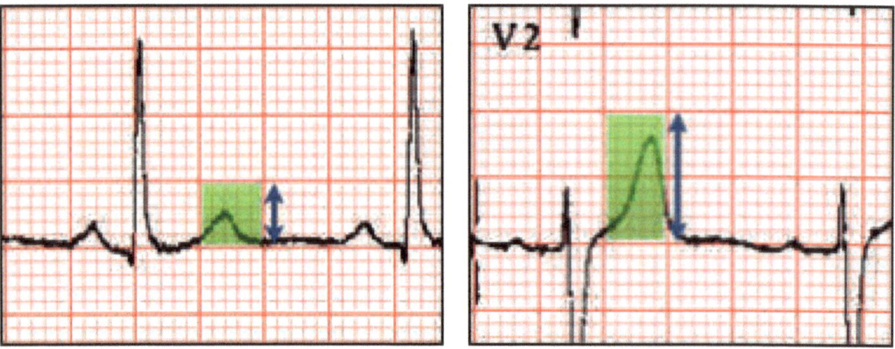

- *QT Interval:* Normally it is less than half of the RR interval

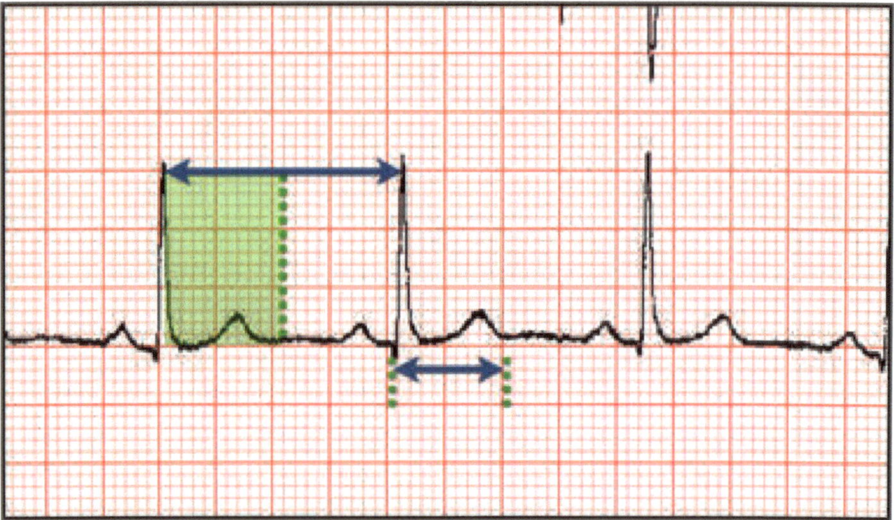

GLOSSARY

Acute coronary syndrome: A condition indicating heart problems due to reduced blood flow to the heart.

Anatomical relationship: The physical location of structures in relation to each other.

Anterior: Referring to the front part of the heart.

Anteroseptal: Pertaining to the front and middle wall of the heart.

Atria: The two upper chambers of the heart.

Atrial fibrillation: An irregular, rapid heart rhythm originating in the atria.

Atrial flutter: A rapid, regular heart rhythm originating in the atria.

Bradyarrhythmia: An abnormally slow heart rhythm.

Bradycardia: A slow heart rate, defined as fewer than 60 beats per minute.

Cardiac: Pertaining to the heart.

Cardiac arrest: A sudden loss of heart function, resulting in the cessation of blood circulation.

Cardiac axis: The direction of the heart's electrical activity.

Calibration: The process of standardizing an ECG machine to ensure accurate readings.

Contiguous: Adjacent or neighboring.

Depolarization: The process of the heart muscle becoming electrically activated and initiating contraction.

ECG: Electrocardiogram, a recording of the heart's electrical activity.

Electrode: A sensor placed on the skin to detect electrical signals from the heart.

Heart rate: The number of times the heart beats per minute.

Hyperkalemia: An abnormally high level of potassium in the blood.

Inferior: Referring to the lower part of the heart.

Lateral: Referring to the side of the heart.

Lead: A specific view or angle of the heart's electrical activity, recorded by combining signals from multiple electrodes.

Myocardial infarction: A heart attack caused by a blockage of blood flow to the heart muscle.

Normal sinus rhythm: A regular heart rhythm originating from the sinoatrial (SA) node, with a rate of 60-100 beats per minute.

Posterior: Referring to the back part of the heart.

Polymorphic ventricular tachycardia: A rapid, irregular heart rhythm originating in the ventricles with changing shapes of the ECG waves.

Precordial leads: Electrodes placed on the chest to record electrical activity.

Repolarization: The process of the heart muscle returning to its resting state after contraction.

Rhythm: The pattern of the heart's electrical activity.

Sinus bradycardia: A slow heart rate originating from the heart's natural pacemaker.

Sinus tachycardia: A fast heart rate originating from the heart's natural pacemaker

Supraventricular tachycardia: A rapid heart rhythm originating above the ventricles.

Tachyarrhythmia: An abnormally rapid heart rhythm.

Tachycardia: An abnormally rapid heart rate, defined as a heart rate above 100 beats per minute.

Ventricles: The two lower chambers of the heart.

Ventricular fibrillation: A chaotic, rapid heart rhythm originating in the ventricles, preventing effective blood pumping.

Ventricular tachycardia: A rapid heart rhythm originating in the ventricles.

INDEX

www.ingramcontent.com/pod-product-compliance
Lightning Source LLC
Chambersburg PA
CBHW040911110726
48005CB00006B/867